Clinical Nutrition

Clinical Nutrition
A PHYSIOLOGIC APPROACH

MEREDITH HOLLOWAY OVERTON, R.D., M.S.
Mead Johnson Laboratories,
Evansville, Indiana

AND

BARBARA P. LUKERT, M.D., F.A.C.P.
Section of Endocrinology and Metabolism,
Department of Medicine,
The University of Kansas Medical Center,
College of Health Sciences and Hospital,
Kansas City, Kansas

YEAR BOOK MEDICAL PUBLISHERS, INC.
CHICAGO • LONDON

Library of Congress Catalog Card Number: 77-81527

International Standard Book Number: 0-8151-5648-0

This book is dedicated to Dr. Sam Roberts and his wife, Mary. Doctor Roberts was on the faculty of the University of Kansas School of Medicine in the Department of Otorhinolaryngology and had a life-long interest in nutrition and nutrition education. Mary Roberts shared his interest and continued to be active in this field after his death.

Preface

"There is not a branch of medicine that does not have some aspect of nutrition within its domain."   H. D. Kruse

THE FIELD OF NUTRITION has survived many shifts in emphasis. During the early 1900s, nutrition was recognized as an area of major importance in medicine. Toward the middle of the century, the development of new drugs, particularly antibiotics, overshadowed advances in nutrition. The past decade has seen a resurgence of interest in this area and the realization that medical school curricula have provided very little information about either preventive or therapeutic nutrition.

This book represents an effort to compile as much clinically useful information as possible and to present it concisely in one source. It is anticipated that the student will consult the references for more detailed accounts.

MEREDITH HOLLOWAY OVERTON
BARBARA P. LUKERT

Page

4 - 5 - 6 - 7 - 8 - 14 - 23 - 36 - 37 - 76 - 90

92 - 94 - 96 - 98 - 99 - 100 ~ 106 ~ 118 - 119 - 120

122 - 124 - 133 ~ 136 - 139 ~ 152 - 154 - 155

156 - 157 ~ 161 - 162

Table of Contents

Chapter 1 / Nutrition and Nutritional Assessment

SCIENTIFIC NUTRITION was born in departments of physiology before they separated from biochemistry. Therefore, many physiologists have retained interest in energy requirements and expenditure. Applied and clinical nutrition were developed in departments of home economics in many colleges and universities but were sorely neglected in medical schools. At the First White House Conference on Food, Nutrition and Health in 1969, the multidisciplinary science of nutrition came of age. The recommendations strongly emphasized the need for greatly improved techniques of educating all relevant professional groups in nutrition and for adequate education of the public in dietary requirements and standards of safety. These recommendations were made after focusing on three major problems: (1) the extent of malnutrition due to poverty in the United States of America; (2) the ignorance of a high proportion of the American population about what constitutes an adequate diet (too many people were "the prey of food faddists and quacks"); and (3) the high content of saturated fats in the national American diet.[59]

In 1972, Bralove reviewed studies of vitamin and mineral nutrition among Americans above poverty status from 1950 to 1968, revealing that "the nutrition of a significant proportion of the American public is inadequate and has become worse during the past 10 years."[8] Approximately 10% of the U.S. population is anemic, while about 25% of Americans are seriously overweight. According to Bralove, "Most people seem to have only a vague understanding of their nutritional needs and the values provided by various foods—and they don't get much help from the medical profession."[8]

Clinical nutrition is intimately bound with the rest of medicine. Modification of the patient's diet is an integral part of the total treatment of diabetes, diverticulosis, pregnancy, obesity, renal disease, coronary heart disease and several gastrointestinal diseases. For all diseases in which diet therapy is significant, certain basic principles of good nutrition should govern the dietary management.[16, 28, 59] "It cannot be assumed that simply because a patient is receiving medical care his nutritional status is thus taken care of automatically. Dietary problems cannot be treated by oversight."[28]

1

Nutritional Assessment

For too long a period, malnutrition has been associated with the "classical" vitamin deficiencies, such as beriberi, scurvy and pellagra. In addition, malnutrition is most often identified with underdeveloped countries, in which incomes and educational levels are low. Kwashiorkor and marasmus have been considered the major nutritional diseases of small children in underdeveloped nations. However, in the past 2 years protein-calorie malnutrition has been found in American hospitals, and it affects one fourth to one half of medical and surgical patients whose hospitalization extended 2 weeks or more.[12] Though it is uncertain whether hospital-induced malnutrition has always been present but only recently has been recognized by nutrition-conscious physicians or whether it has become an unexpected byproduct of sophisticated food service systems in our institutions, hospital malnutrition is a prevalent professional and legal health problem.

It is important that physicians, nurses and hospital administrators, as well as dietitians, become aware of the nutritional status of hospitalized patients. Good nutrition plays a major role in wound healing and resistance to infection. Nutritional support can be provided to the patient through various new products and techniques; so there is no real reason why a patient cannot be adequately nourished. Nutritional assessment of the patient is every health care professional's responsibility.

Nutritional assessment generally has four components: anthropometric measurements, clinical assessment, biochemical assessment and dietary methodologies. To evaluate the nutritional status of a group of people in a specified community, a fifth component—community assessment (background information)—is added. Anthropometric measurements generally include height and weight, skin fold measurements (triceps, subscapular or midaxillary), arm circumference, upper arm muscle diameter and head circumference (especially in infants and children). Clinical assessment consists of the patient's history and physical examination. Certain physical signs, such as easily plucked hair or pale conjunctivae, are indicative or suggestive of malnutrition. Biochemical assessment may encompass common laboratory tests, such as serum albumin and a complete blood count, and/or functional laboratory tests, such as fecal fat and D-xylose tolerance test. Dietary methodologies are used to determine an individual's dietary or nutritional intake and to assess the need for intervention or correction. These determinations may be obtained through 24-hour

TABLE 1-1.–SIGNS USED IN NUTRITION SURVEYS RECOMMENDED BY THE WHO REPORT OF EXPERT COMMITTEE ON MEDICAL ASSESSMENT OF NUTRITIONAL STATUS*

AREA OF EXAMI- NATION	GROUP 1: SIGNS KNOWN TO BE OF VALUE IN NUTRITION SURVEYS	GROUP 2: SIGNS THAT NEED FURTHER INVESTIGATION	GROUP 3: SOME SIGNS NOT RELATED TO NUTRITION
1. Hair	Lack of luster Thinness and sparseness Depigmentation of proximal part of hair Flag sign Easy pluckability of hair		Alopecia Artificial discoloration
2. Face	Diffuse depigmentation Nasolabial dyssebacea Moon face	Malar and supraocular pigmentation	Acne vulgaris Acne rosacea Chloasma
3. Eyes	Xerosis conjunctivae Xerophthalmia (including keratomalacia) Bitot's spots Blepharitis angularis	Conjunctival infection Circumcorneal infection Circumcorneal and scleral pigmentation Corneal vascularization Corneal opacities and scars	Follicular conjunctivitis Blepharitis Pingueculae Pterygium Pannus
4. Lips	Angular stomatitis Angular scars Cheilosis	Chronic depigmentation of lower lip	Chapping from exposure to harsh climates
5. Tongue	Edema Scarlet and raw tongue Magenta tongue Atrophic papillae	Hyperemic and hypertrophic papillae Fissures Geographic tongue Pigmented tongue	Aphthous ulcer Leukoplakia
6. Teeth	Mottled enamel	Caries Attrition Enamel hypoplasia Enamel erosion	Malocclusion
7. Gums	Spongy, bleeding gums	Recession of gum	Pyorrhea
8. Glands	Thyroid enlargement Parotid enlargement	Gynecomastia	Allergic or inflammatory enlargement of thyroid or parotid

*From Isaksson, B.[35]

recall, dietary records, history of foods eaten over a long period of time or self-administered questionnaire for general dietary data or information on specific foods.[12, 13, 32, 35]

In the progression of clinical undernutrition, a gradual tissue desaturation of nutrients and biochemical lesions precede anatomical lesions and signs of deficiency. Therefore, absence of physical signs

TABLE 1-2.—VITAMINS AND THEIR BIOCHEMICAL ACTION

VITAMIN	BIOCHEMICAL ACTION	RESULT OF VITAMIN DEFICIENCY
Thiamine (B_1)	1. Coenzyme catalyzing decarboxylation of pyruvic acid and α-ketoglutaric acid	Anorexia, peripheral neuropathy, heart failure
	2. Transketolase reaction	Beriberi
Riboflavin (B_2)	1. Flavoprotein enzyme system	Scaly skin, weight loss, cheilosis, weakness
	2. As coenzyme in: amino acid demethylase, monoamino oxidase, xanthine oxidase, glutathione reductase	
Niacin	1. Constituent of respiratory coenzyme NAD	Pellagra
	2. Codehydrogenase for metabolism of lactate, alcohol and β-hydroxybutyrate	Dermatitis, diarrhea, dementia, death
Pyridoxine (B_6)	1. Coenzyme for transaminases, decarboxylases, deaminases, desulfurases	Anemia, seizures, peripheral neuropathy
Folic acid	Coenzyme:	
	1. Transfer of single carbon units	Megaloblastic anemia, neuropathy
	2. Thymidine synthesis	
	3. Hydroxylation reactions	
B_{12}	1. Transmethylation	Megaloblastic anemia, glossitis, achlorhydria, posterior spinal column degeneration
	2. Methyl biosynthesis	
	3. Disulfide reduction	
	4. Activation of folic acid coenzymes	
C	1. Antioxidant-reducing substance	Bleeding gums, petechiae hyperkeratotic hair follicles, rarefaction of bone, poor wound healing
	2. Hydroxylation of proline tryptophan	
	3. Iron reduction	
A	1. Cell membrane stability	Dry skin, night blindness, follicular hyperkeratosis; xerophthalmia, Bitot's spots
	2. Mucopolysaccharide formation	
	3. Formation of visual pigments	
D	1. Increases calcium and phosphorus absorption from intestine	Rickets in children, osteomalacia in adults
	2. Initiates calcification	
K	1. Catalyzes synthesis of prothrombin	Hemorrhage
	2. Cofactor for oxidative phosphorylation	
E	1. Antioxidant	None recognized

does not rule out malnutrition. Table 1–1 describes signs used in nutrition surveys recommended by the World Health Organization (WHO) Report of the Expert Committee on Medical Assessment of Nutritional Status.[35] Signs indicative of protein-calorie malnutrition are edema, depigmentation and easy pluckability of the hair; thin, sparse hair; muscle wasting; moon face, hepatomegaly; and flaky-paint dermatosis. Xerosis conjunctivae, Bitot's spots and xerosis corneae are signs of vitamin A deficiency. Vitamin B complex deficiency may be indicated by angular stomatitis, cheilosis, glossitis, atrophic lingual papillae and hypertrophic lingual papillae. The presence of only one of these signs could justify suspicion of undernutrition and need for further investigation.[35] The role of vitamins in metabolic pathways and the result of vitamin deficiencies can be found in Table 1–2.

In assessment of the vitamin status of an individual, thiamine, riboflavin and N-1-methylnicotinamide in the urine can be measured; for folic acid, the content of serum can be determined by radioimmunoassay; and for vitamin D, by radiologic investigation of the skeleton and in some centers measurement of 25-hydroxycholecalciferol level. The results of many of these tests are influenced by various factors. Therefore, one should not rely on a single test in borderline cases.[10] Table 1–3 lists special laboratory tests that can be used in nutritional assessment. It should be kept in mind that drugs, vitamins, antibiotics, con-

TABLE 1–3.—SPECIAL LABORATORY TESTS OF VALUE IN NUTRITIONAL ASSESSMENT°

NUTRIENT AND UNITS	AGE OF SUBJECT (YEARS)	DEFICIENT	CRITERIA OF STATUS MARGINAL	ACCEPT-ABLE
Serum ascorbic acid (mg/100 ml)†	All ages	Up to 0.1	0.1–0.19	0.2+
Plasma vitamin A (μg/100 ml)†	All ages	Up to 10	10–19	20+
Plasma carotene (μg/100 ml)†	All ages	Up to 20	20–39	40+
	Pregnant	–	40–79	80+
Serum folacin (ng/ml)‡	All ages	Up to 2.0	2.1–5.9	6.0+
Serum vitamin B₁₂ (pg/ml)‡	All ages	Up to 100	–	100+
Thiamine in urine (μg/gm creatinine)†	1–3	Up to 120	120–175	175+
	4–5	Up to 85	85–120	120+
	6–9	Up to 70	70–180	180+
	10–15	Up to 55	55–150	150+
	16+	Up to 27	27–65	65+
	Pregnant	Up to 21	21–49	50+

(continued)

TABLE 1-3.—*Continued*

Riboflavin in urine (µg/gm creatinine)†	1-3	Up to 150	150-499	500+
	4-5	Up to 100	100-299	300+
	6-9	Up to 85	85-269	270+
	10-16	Up to 70	70-199	200+
	16+	Up to 27	27-79	80+
	Pregnant	Up to 30	30-89	90+
RBC transketo-lase-TPP-effect (ratio)‡	All ages	25+	15-25	Up to 15
RBC glutathione reductase-FAD-effect (ratio)‡	All ages	1.2+	—	Up to 1.2
Tryptophan load (mg xanthurenic acid excreted)‡	Adults (dose: 100 mg/kg body weight)	25 + (6 hr) 75 + (24 hr)	— —	Up to 25 Up to 75
Urinary pyridoxine (µg/gm creatinine)‡	1-3	Up to 90	—	90+
	4-6	Up to 80	—	80+
	7-9	Up to 60	—	60+
	10-12	Up to 40	—	40+
	13-15	Up to 30	—	30+
	16+	Up to 20	—	20+
Urinary N-1-methyl-nicotinamide (mg/gm creatinine)†	All ages Pregnant	Up to 0.2 Up to 0.8	0.2-5.59 0.8-2.49	0.6+ 2.5+
Urinary pantothenic acid (µg)‡	All ages	Up to 200	—	200+
Plasma vitamin E (mg/100 ml)‡	All ages	Up to 0.2	0.2-0.6	0.6+

*From Butterworth, C. E., and Blackburn, G. L.[12] Derived from Table of Current Guidelines for Criteria of Nutritional Status for Laboratory Evaluation, in Christakis, G. (ed.): Nutritional assessment in health programs, Am. J. Public Health (suppl.) 63:34, 1973. Also see Sauberlich, H. E., Dowdy, R. P., and Skala, J. H.: Laboratory tests for the assessment of nutritional status, CRC Crit. Rev. Clin. Lab. Sci. 4:215, 1973.
†Adapted from the Ten State Nutrition Survey.
‡Criteria may vary with different methodology.

traceptive steroids and other agents may influence the outcome of some laboratory studies.[12]

To assess the nutritional status of a patient in the hospital, the physician should review promptly all nutrition-related information provided by various staff members and correlate it with his own observations, physical findings and preliminary laboratory data. He should itemize the specific nutrition problems on the problem list in front of the patient's record. The history, physical examination and laboratory findings comprise the physician's tools for nutritional assessment. Table 1-4 is a checklist for assessment of nutritional status by several health care team members. The accurate recordings of the patient's

TABLE 1-4.—CHECKLIST FOR ASSESSMENT OF NUTRITIONAL STATUS°

Part 1
(To be completed by trained staff member, physician's assistant or other)

Usual body weight 20% above or below desirable?
Recent loss or gain of 10% of usual body weight?
Any evidence that income and meals are not adequate for needs?
More than half of meals eaten away from home?
Does patient live alone and prepare own meals?
Ill-fitting dentures?
Excessive use of alcohol?
Frequent use of fad diets or monotonous diets?
Any chronic disease of GI tract? (Describe)
Has there been any surgical procedure on GI tract (other than appendectomy)?
  (Describe)
Recent major surgery, illness or injury?
Recent use of large doses of:
  Catabolic steroids?
  Immunosuppressants?
  Antitumor agents?
  Anticonvulsants?
  Antibiotics?
  Oral contraceptives?
  Vitamins?
  Other?
Has patient been maintained more than 10 days on intravenous fluids?
Any reason to anticipate that patient will be unable to eat for 10 days or longer?
Is patient known to have:
  Diabetes?
  Hypertension?
  Hyperlipidemia?
  Coronary artery disease?
  Malabsorption?
  Chronic lung disease?
  Chronic renal disease?
  Chronic liver disease?
  Circulatory problem or heart failure?
  Neurologic disorder or paralysis?
  Mental retardation?

(Note: If all answers to the above items are "No," the patient may be regarded as a "low-risk" or "acceptable risk." The risk increases in direct proportion to the number of "Yes" answers. Patients with more than 3 "Yes" answers should be considered at an increased risk of developing medical complications, unless special attention is given to providing their nutritional requirements.)

Part 2
(To be completed by dietitian)

Description of recent food consumption patterns, eating habits and meal composition.
Circumstances of food purchase, storage and preparation in the home.
Estimate of daily average caloric consumption.
Estimate of energy expenditure (e.g., low, average or high level of physical activity).
Estimate of possible nutrient deficiencies, based on suspected imbalances.
Food tray viewed.   *(continued)*

TABLE 1-4.—*Continued*

Part 3
(To be completed by nursing staff)

Estimate of actual food consumption, including any provided by nonhospital sources.
Estimate of fluid intake.
Estimate of stool frequency, urinary losses, losses by suction tube, drainage, etc.
Behavior patterns, eccentricities, vomiting (including surreptitious vomiting).
Careful recording of body weight at regular intervals.

°From Butterworth, C. E. and Blackburn, G. L.[12]

height and weight are just as imperative as the recording of prescribed medications. Whenever a patient is suspected of becoming malnourished, observations made by the dietitian and nurses regarding his meal trays are of great importance and should be documented for the physician's awareness.[12]

In May 1974, three single-day nutritional surveys were conducted at weekly intervals in the general medical wards of an urban municipal teaching hospital. Anthropometric measures (weight/height, triceps skin fold and arm muscle circumference) and biochemical measures (serum albumin, hematocrit and percent of lymphocytes) were the methods of nutritional assessment. The patient's nutrient intake from the previous week was classified according to the likelihood of meeting daily protein and calorie requirements. The prevalence of protein-calorie malnutrition was 44% or greater. A similar survey of surgical patients disclosed that in comparison the medical patients had better protein status (arm muscle circumference, serum albumin) but were more depleted calorically (weight/height, triceps skin fold). Nonetheless, protein-calorie malnutrition exists quite frequently in municipal hospitals among patients on medical and surgical services.[4]

Butterworth and Blackburn described three categories of malnutrition. The first was the "adult kwashiorkor-like state," which evolved from a protein-deficient diet. Patients in an adult kwashiorkor-like state maintained their anthropometric measurements despite severe depression of serum proteins, transferrin and albumin. Edema and the depression of cellular immune function, which was measured by lymphocyte counts, humoral and leukocyte competence and delayed hypersensitivity skin testing, were common.[12]

The second type of protein-calorie malnutrition was "adult marasmus or chronic inanition," which was characterized by decreased anthropometric measurements and normal serum albumin. This prolonged and gradual wasting of muscle mass and subcutaneous fat was due to inadequate intake of protein and calories. The "marasmic kwashiorkor-like state" was the third category of malnutrition. It was regarded as an advanced state, combined some of the clinical features of the other two types and was signaled by the onset of hypoalbuminemia, edema, depressed immunologic competence and evidence of deterioration in the function of multiple organ systems. Thus, the marasmic kwashiorkor-like state is life-threatening and requires more urgent and complex care.[12]

In 1974, Butterworth referred to iatrogenic malnutrition as an euphemism for "physician-induced malnutrition" and believed that the inevitable consequences of the lack of nutrition education in medical schools were being seen. Physicians tend to overlook a patient's nutrition and treat only the initial complaint. Although it is well known that malnutrition interferes with wound healing and increases susceptibility to infection, malnutrition is rarely considered by some physicians and surgeons as contributing to mortality, morbidity and prolonged bed-occupancy rates. Protein, zinc and vitamin C are essentials for wound healing but may often be depleted in a postsurgical patient who has not been eating because of a poor appetite or an improperly advanced diet. Further, certain drugs given to hospitalized patients, such as aspirin, barbiturates and diphenylhydantoin, increase vitamin C and folate requirements.[11]

In concluding, Butterworth listed 14 undesirable practices that can affect the nutritional health of hospitalized patients: (1) Failure to record height and weight. (2) Frequent rotation of staff. (3) Diffusion of responsibility for patient care. (4) Prolonged intravenous feedings of glucose and saline. (5) Failure to observe patients' food intake. (6) Meals withheld because of diagnostic tests. (7) Tube feedings in inadequate amounts, of uncertain composition and under unsanitary conditions. (8) Ignorance of the composition of vitamin mixtures and other nutritional products. (9) Failure to recognize increased nutritional needs due to injury or illness. (10) Failure to ascertain whether the patient is optimally nourished before surgery and inadequate nutritional support after surgery. (11) Failure to appreciate the role of nutrition in the prevention of and recovery from infection, with an unwarranted reliance on antibiotics. (12) Lack of communication and interaction between physician and dietitian. (As staff professionals, dietitians should be concerned with the nutritional health of *every* patient.) (13) Delay of nutritional support until a patient is in an advanced state of depletion, which is sometimes irreversible. (14) Limited availability of laboratory tests to assess nutritional status or failure to use those that are available.[11]

From the reports and discussion in the literature came the *Manual for Nutritional/Metabolic Assessment of the Hospitalized Patient*, which was presented at the 62d Annual Clinical Congress of the American College of Surgeons in Chicago, October 1976, by George L. Blackburn, M.D., and his associates. The manual stated that an awareness of the nutritional/metabolic status of the hospitalized patient is essential for all patient care personnel. The manual contains charts, tables and graphs that health care professionals can use to determine mid-upper arm circumference and triceps skin fold, ideal weight, creatinine/height index, estimated energy expenditure and oxygen consumption, body urea nitrogen losses, categories of clinically significant changes in malnutrition and hypermetabolism and rates of nutritional depletion. The manual also provides examples of a patient nutritional assessment form, nutrition/metabolic profile for computer use, computer printout sheet for comprehensive nutrition/metabolic profile and others.[5] If only used in part, this material should prove useful in assessing a patient's nutritional status, but much of the information would prove useful only in clinical studies.

Infant Nutrition

The early months of life constitute the period of most rapid growth in childhood or at any time of life. During this period, the brain and central nervous system develop rapidly, and the supply of essential nutrients is crucial for normal development. The energy requirement per unit of body weight is much greater for infants than for any other age group. For instance, energy requirements for basal metabolism alone are 25 kcal/lb body weight each day. Generally during the first six months, an infant's total energy requirement per day is 50–55 kcal/lb or 117 kcal/kg. From six months to one year, the infant's total energy requirement is reduced slightly to 40–45 kcal/lb or 108

TABLE 1–5.—DETERMINATION OF AMOUNT OF FORMULA TO BE FED TO AN INFANT WITHIN 24 HOURS

AGE	ENERGY REQUIREMENT (KCAL/LB)	KCAL/OZ OF FORMULA	OZ OF FORMULA/LB
0–6 mo	50–55	20	2.5–2.75
6 mo–1 yr	40–45	20	2.0–2.25
Premature infant for first year	55–60	24	2.3–2.5

Total amount of formula for 24 hours = infant's weight in lb × amount of formula/lb
Example—an 8-lb infant, aged 0–2 months:
8 lb × 2.5 oz formula/lb = 20 oz formula/24 hr

kcal/kg each day. Table 1-5 shows how to calculate the amount of formula necessary to supply these energy requirements for 24 hours. Protein requirements for growth and development are greater during infancy, which means an infant requires 1.0-1.5 gm protein/lb body weight, or, as the recommended daily dietary allowances (RDA) state, 2.2 gm protein/kg body weight for the first six months and 2.0 gm protein/kg from six months to one year (Table 1-6). A major source of calories (50% or more) in the infant's diet is fat, which supplies the arachidonic and linoleic acids essential for normal cell formation.

To maintain an adequate rate of growth and proper utilization of the carbohydrates, protein and fat, a continuous supply of vitamins, minerals and trace elements, such as zinc, copper, and magnesium, is needed. Rapid rate of growth and little, if any, body stores of some of these nutrients make the dietary supply of them vital. The rate and extent of cellular multiplication and tissue maturation are solely dependent upon the infant's diet.

Generally, it takes six months to a year (more like the latter) for the gastrointestinal tract and kidneys to develop fully. Therefore, it is important to supply adequate nutrition without stressing these systems. Large proteins, such as those from cow's milk, pass through the intestine without significant digestion and absorption. This may be important when considering mechanisms in the development of allergies. Excess dietary nitrogen from proteins form greater amounts of urea, which eventually is excreted through the kidneys, along with excess sodium, chloride and potassium. Excretion of large solute loads requires extra water from body fluid reserves, which can reduce the margin of safety for water losses associated with diarrhea. Consequently, a low renal solute load helps maintain body fluid homeostasis and protects against renal overload. Since total body water by weight in an infant is about 80%, maintenance of high water content in the formula is vital to offset the usual high evaporative water losses. Human milk can maintain adequate fluid reserves by its particular concentration of water and solids.[26]

As Townley stated, "Although breast feeding still seems the most desirable means of infant feeding, it is obvious that many mothers, for various reasons, prefer to feed their babies artificially."[60] The nutrient content of breast milk provides a total diet which balances the requirements for normal growth and development while reducing the stress associated with digestion, metabolism and excretion. However, the most desirable alternative is infant formula patterned after breast milk. Only 20% of infants are breast-fed during the first month of life,

CLINICAL NUTRITION

TABLE 1-6.—FOOD AND NUTRITION BOARD
RESEARCH COUNCIL RECOMMENDED
Designed for the maintenance of good nutrition

	AGE (yr)	WEIGHT (kg)	WEIGHT (lb)	HEIGHT (cm)	HEIGHT (in.)	ENERGY (kcal)†	PROTEIN (gm)	FAT-SOLUBLE VITAMINS			
								VITA-MIN A ACTIVITY (RE)‡	(IU)	VITA-MIN D (IU)	VITA-MIN E ACTIVITY‖ (IU)
Infants	0.0–0.5	6	14	60	24	kg × 117	kg × 2.2	420§	1,400	400	4
	0.5–1.0	9	20	71	28	kg × 108	kg × 2.0	400	2,000	400	5
Children	1–3	13	28	86	34	1,300	23	400	2,000	400	7
	4–6	20	44	110	44	1,800	30	500	2,500	400	9
	7–10	30	66	135	54	2,400	36	700	3,300	400	10
Males	11–14	44	97	158	63	2,800	44	1,000	5,000	400	12
	15–18	61	134	172	69	3,000	54	1,000	5,000	400	15
	19–22	67	147	172	69	3,000	54	1,000	5,000	400	15
	23–50	70	154	172	69	2,700	56	1,000	5,000		15
	51+	70	154	172	69	2,400	56	1,000	5,000		15
Females	11–14	44	97	155	62	2,400	44	800	4,000	400	12
	15–18	54	119	162	65	2,100	48	800	4,000	400	12
	19–22	58	128	162	65	2,100	46	800	4,000	400	12
	23–50	58	128	162	65	2,000	46	800	4,000		12
	51+	58	128	162	65	1,800	46	800	4,000		12
Pregnant						+300	+30	1,000	5,000	400	15
Lactating						+500	+20	1,200	6,000	400	15

*The allowances are intended to provide for individual variations among most normal persons as they live in the United States under usual environmental stresses. Diets should be based on a variety of common foods in order to provide other nutrients for which human requirements have been less well defined.
†Kilojoules (kJ) = 4.2 × kcal.
‡Retinol equivalents.
§Assumed to be all as retinol in milk during the first six months of life. All subsequent intakes are assumed to be half as retinol and half as β-carotene when calculated from international units. As retinol equivalents, three fourths are as retinol and one fourth as β-carotene.
‖Total vitamin E activity, estimated to be 80% as α-tocopherol and 20% other tocopherols. See text for variation in allowances.
¶The folacin allowances refer to dietary sources as determined by *Lactobacillus casei* assay. Pure forms of folacin may be effective in doses less than one fourth of the recommended dietary allowance.
**Although allowances are expressed as niacin, it is recognized that on the average 1 mg niacin is derived from each 60 mg dietary tryptophan.
††This increased requirement cannot be met by ordinary diets; therefore, the use of supplemental iron is recommended.

while 64% are fed milk-based formulas. By the fifth month, only 5% of infants are breast-fed, while 29% are fed milk-based formulas. Less than 2% of infants are fed either breast milk or milk-based formula by nine months.[30] Although these figures are decreasing, the percentage of infants fed cow's milk is increasing. Modern living has caused infants to adopt adult habits and patterns of food consumption too early. The percentage of calories provided by solid foods progressively increases from 30% at 2–3 months to 40% at 5–6 months, and 66% at 9–12 months.[30]

The composition of breast milk and comparable commercially available infant formula can be compared to cow's milk, the earliest substitution made in an infant's diet. Keep in mind the review of gastrointestinal tract and kidney development in the infant. In human milk, 7% of the calories is protein, 42% is carbohydrate and 51% is fat. In-

NATIONAL ACADEMY OF SCIENCES-NATIONAL DAILY DIETARY ALLOWANCES,* REVISED 1974[53]
of practically all healthy people in the U.S.A.

ASCOR-BIC ACID (mg)	FOLA-CIN¶ (μg)	NIA-CIN** (mg)	RIBO-FLAVIN (mg)	THIA-MIN (mg)	VITA-MIN B_6 (mg)	VITA-MIN B_{12} (μg)	CAL-CIUM (mg)	PHOS-PHORUS (mg)	IODINE (μg)	IRON (mg)	MAG-NESIUM (mg)	ZINC (mg)
35	50	5	0.4	0.3	0.3	0.3	360	240	35	10	60	3
35	50	8	0.6	0.5	0.4	0.3	540	400	45	15	70	5
40	100	9	0.8	0.7	0.6	1.0	800	800	60	15	150	10
40	200	12	1.1	0.9	0.9	1.5	800	800	80	10	200	10
40	300	16	1.2	1.2	1.2	2.0	800	800	110	10	250	10
45	400	18	1.5	1.4	1.6	3.0	1,200	1,200	130	18	350	15
45	400	20	1.8	1.5	2.0	3.0	1,200	1,200	150	18	400	15
45	400	20	1.8	1.5	2.0	3.0	800	800	140	10	350	15
45	400	18	1.6	1.4	2.0	3.0	800	800	130	10	350	15
45	400	16	1.5	1.2	2.0	3.0	800	800	110	10	350	15
45	400	16	1.3	1.2	1.6	3.0	1,200	1,200	115	18	300	15
45	400	14	1.4	1.1	2.0	3.0	1,200	1,200	115	18	300	15
45	400	14	1.4	1.1	2.0	3.0	800	800	100	18	300	15
45	400	13	1.2	1.0	2.0	3.0	800	800	100	18	300	15
45	400	12	1.1	1.0	2.0	3.0	800	800	80	10	300	15
60	800	+2	+0.3	+0.3	2.5	4.0	1,200	1,200	125	18+††	450	20
80	600	+4	+0.5	+0.3	2.5	4.0	1,200	1,200	150	18	450	25

fant formulas have been processed to contain similar amounts of these three major nutrients: Enfamil contains 9% protein, 41% carbohydrate and 50% fat; Similac contains 11% protein, 41% carbohydrate and 48% fat; and S-M-A contains 9% protein, 43% carbohydrate and 48% fat. In comparison, whole cow's milk contains 22% protein, 30% carbohydrate and 48% fat. In addition to the great variation in protein content, the mineral and vitamin content of cow's milk is unsatisfactory for infants; cow's milk contains too much calcium, phosphorus, sodium and potassium and too little iron, vitamin C, vitamin E, etc. For a more complete comparison, see Table 1–7.

The Committee on Nutrition of the American Academy of Pediatrics has written and updated, in 1976, some proposed standards for infant formulas. Recommendations for caloric density, osmolarity, reconstitution, protein content, fat and essential fatty acids, carbohydrate, vita-

TABLE 1-7.—COMPARISON OF NUTRIENT COMPOSITION PER QUART

	ENFAMIL	BREAST MILK	WHOLE MILK§	SKIM MILK	2% MILK	SIMILAC	S-M-A
Calories, kcal	640	670	634	354	590	640	640
Protein, gm	14.2	11.0	34.0	35.4	42.0	15.5	14.4
Fat, gm	35.0	43.0	34.0	1.0	20.0	36.1	34.6
Carbohydrate, gm	66.2	64.0	48.0	51.0	60.5	72.3	69.1
Caloric distribution							
Protein, % cal	9	7	22	40	28	11	9
Fat, % cal	50	51	48	3	31	48	48
Carbohydrate, % cal	41	42	30	57	41	41	43
Vitamin A, IU	1600	1660	1366	Trace	800	1365	2500
Vitamin D, IU	400	4	400	12‡	235‡	378	400
Vitamin E, IU	12	6	1.4	Trace†	1.7†	8.5	9
Vitamin C, mg	50	43	10	10	10	52	55
Folic acid, μg	100	25	2	2	2.5	47	30
Thiamine, mg	0.5	0.2	0.29	0.39	0.40	0.061	0.067
Riboflavin, mg	0.4	0.4	1.66	1.77	2.10	0.095	1
Niacin, mg	8	1.5	9	9	11.20	6.6	9.5
Vitamin B_6, mg	0.4	0.1	0.5	0.5	0.6	0.038	0.4
Vitamin B_{12}, μg	2	Trace	5	5†	6†	1.4	1
Pantothenic acid, mg	3	1.8	3	3†	3.7†	2.8	2
Vitamin K, μg	66–100	14.2	57	57	57	–	55
Choline, mg	85	85	120	125†	148†	–	–
Calcium, mg	520	320	1150	1192	1430	660	420
Phosphorus, mg	440	140	920	936	1120	520	312
Iodine, μg	65	30	200	208	250	39	65
Iron, mg	1.4*	1.4	Trace	Trace	Trace	Trace‖	12
Magnesium, mg	45	40	120	34†	150†	39	50
Copper, mg	0.6	0.03	0.3	0.3	0.4	0.39	0.4
Zinc, mg	4	5	3.6	3.6	3.6	–	–
Manganese, mg	1	0.01	Trace	Trace	Trace	–	–
Potassium, mg	660	530	1405	1427	1750	795	530
Sodium, mg	265	145	488	512	610	310	142

*Enfamil with iron contains 12 mg/quart.
†Calculated in proportion to the protein level.
‡Calculated in proportion to the fat level.
§Fortified with 400 IU of Vitamin D per quart.
‖Similac with iron contains 12 mg/quart.
References: Newer Knowledge of Milk, (National Dairy Council, 1965) and Milk: The Mammary Gland and Its Secretion (1961).

mins (niacin, vitamin B_6, vitamin A, vitamin D, vitamin K, vitamin E, biotin, choline and inositol amended) and minerals (changes made for sodium, potassium, chloride, calcium, phosphorus, iron, zinc, copper and manganese) are presented. Quoting the Committee, "When breast-feeding is unsuccessful, inappropriate or stopped early, infant formulas provide the best alternative for meeting nutritional needs during the first year."[20]

Overfeeding during infancy is a problem which many investigators have been researching. Maslansky and his associates studied the infant feeding practices of 451 infants from low-income families in New York. Half the infants were started on solid foods in the first month, and solid foods contributed nearly 40% of the daily calories by four months. Average caloric intakes were 10% above the RDA for infants under six months and 14% above the RDA for infants 6–12 months of age. The average daily protein intake was 62% above the RDA for infants under six months and 105% above the RDA for infants 6–12 months. Dietary iron *insufficiency* tended to increase with increasing age. Daily iron intake averaged only 80% of the RDA for infants under seven months and only 55% of the RDA for infants 6–12 months of age.[42] Purvis estimated that an infant at 13 months had an average daily iron intake of only one-half the RDA.[52] The greatest problem evidenced by these studies, however, was overnutrition.

It is believed that weight gain in infancy reflects an interaction of genetic potential and environmental influences.[38] In recent years, a marked increase of obese infants in the United States has been thought to be related to excessive caloric intake. The old adage, "a fat baby is a healthy baby," is not supported by medical or scientific evidence on withstanding infection and preventing undue stress.[37] In addition, there is a positive association between obese children and obese adults showing increased adiposity.[56] Knittle found that two periods are critical in the development of fat cells: from birth to 2 years and from 8 to 12 years. The number of fat cells is fixed between the ages of 16 and 21.[37] Obviously, the first period influences the rest of one's life.

The infant's large salt intake has reflected the use of salt in solid foods, such as presalted cereals, meats and vegetables.[24] Dahl demonstrated in epidemiologic studies that diets high in salt may induce hypertension. He has hypothesized that infants may be more susceptible than adults.[23] However, genetic predisposition is the most significant factor.[23] In support of this hypothesis, the Committee on Nutrition of the American Academy of Pediatrics has commented, "There is a reasonable possibility that a low salt intake begun early in life may protect, to some extent, persons at risk from developing hypertension."[21]

The pathogenesis of atherosclerosis and coronary heart disease may stem from early life, and these diseases are influenced by dietary reduction of cholesterol, saturated fat and total fat. These factors have led many physicians to recognize the conditions as pediatric problems.[3, 6] Currently, the risk is recognized in infancy only when it is extremely high due to heredity and the infant shows definitive signs. Preventive measures in infancy may play a significant role in retarding the progression of these conditions. Most of the commercial infant formulas contain vegetable fats with a stated polyunsaturated to saturated fat (P/S) ratio.

Nutrition during Childhood

The RDA for children shows three divisions by age. In addition, the energy and protein requirements are no longer in terms of so much per kg body weight but are stated in total amounts. The increases in nutrient requirements tend to level off after the first year of age and show only a small change from 4 through 6 years of age, reflecting the slower rate of growth and development during this period. The increases from 7 through 10 years of age are still slight in comparison to the first year of life and the spurt that comes with adolescence.

Dugdale studied childhood growth and nutrition by taking anthropometric data from three groups of children. These data were analyzed, and similar patterns were found in all groups. Growth of bones and muscles correlated, but the amount of subcutaneous fat varied independently. Three hypotheses were supported by the data:

1. The level of effective protein intake, the protein available after energy needs have been met, is the principal factor controlling growth in height and of muscle bulk. (Development of the central nervous system is also dependent upon early intake of an effective level of protein.)

2. The level of caloric intake is the principal factor controlling the amount of subcutaneous fat.

3. Genetic factors set a ceiling on growth in height but become effective only when nutritional and other factors have reached an optimal level.[27]

Findings from the ten-state nutrition survey of 1968–70 contributed more information on nutrition and growth than had been anticipated. The results pointed out some major gaps in knowledge of this area and provided new but substantive information. "Pot-bellied, spider-limbed malnutrition" was not found nor was the prevalence of "hunger" as presented in a 1967 television documentary. However, the dimensions of poverty could be spelled out in "smaller size" and "lesser growth." Economic level, size and growth do interact with each other in blacks and in whites; and socioeconomics is a relevant factor as an antecedent of obesity.[31]

The American Academy of Pediatrics issued a statement in 1972 on coronary heart disease and the childhood diet. The Committee on Nutrition did not support the Commission for Heart Disease Resources' recommendation for dietary intervention for all children. Trials should be performed on persons with the familial type II defect to determine safety, acceptability and effectiveness of modified diet approach in children. Results of trials should be made available before recommending dietary intervention for *all* children. Dietary cholesterol should be kept as low as possible for children from 1 to 12 years of age with type II hyperlipoproteinemia, but there is "no good reason for initiating the diet before one year of age. . . ."[19] The diet should ensure that food constituents essential to normal growth are provided in adequate quantities. Families with no evidence of type II hyperlipoproteinemia need only be advised that no harm is known to arise from moderate dietary alteration.[19]

Adolescent Nutrition

Adolescence is the second period of rapid growth in life. Changes in height and in the size and function of many glands occur during this period. The amounts of essential amino acids *must* be adequate, and calories must be sufficient for energy requirements. Stunted growth and lack of hair and nail growth are manifestations of protein-calorie malnutrition during this period.[15]

According to Breeling and Mongeau, the nutrients most consistently below 2/3 of the RDA for teenagers are iron, calcium, ascorbic acid and vitamin A.[9, 44] Breeling attributes this undernutrition to the characteristic eating patterns of the teen: frequent eating and snacking, consuming vegetables least regularly, one fifth to one fourth taking vitamin pills and abandoning structured meals in many cases.[9]

Nutrition education often fails with this age group for several reasons. First, teenagers have often been subjected to the dictum "Eat what you don't like because it's good for you." Second, most adolescents do not experience signs or symptoms of malnutrition that adults have warned them will result from their poor eating habits. Third, eating is only one part of the busy lives of teenagers and may often take a back seat to other activities and interests, such as sports and dates. So, what food they need is not always available to them at the proper place and time. Last but not least, persons in the prime positions to help them fail to become knowledgeable themselves.[9]

Adolescence is a difficult period in life for the youngster as well as his parents. Poor nutrition is only one of the problems to be faced, but it certainly is an important one that should be corrected for a healthy future.

Nutrition during Pregnancy

Past studies of nutrition in women during pregnancy have shown a definite relationship between the diet of the mother and the condition of the baby at birth. Some of the complications of pregnancy, such as anemia, toxemia and premature delivery, have been found to result in part from diets that do not meet the nutritional needs of the mother and fetus. A mother who has always eaten a diet adequate in all the essential nutrients and who is in good health has a much better chance of delivering a healthy baby. It has been said that "nutrition for pregnancy begins before conception." This is especially true for the teenage mother, since teenage girls consume diets low in calcium and vitamin D, as well as iron.

When reviewing the nutritional requirements of pregnant women, certain "rules" concerning weight gain should be kept in mind:

Weight of baby	7.50 lb
Weight of placenta	1.25 lb
Increased weight in uterus	3.50 lb
Weight of amniotic fluid	2.50 lb
Increase in weight of breasts	0.75 lb
Increase in blood volume and extracellular fluid	8.50 lb
	————
Total weight	24.00 lb

This total weight gain should be distributed by an increase of ½ lb/week until the 36th week of pregnancy and 1 lb/week from the 36th week forward.[48] Pregnancy is not the time to reduce the overweight patient. Severe calorie restriction is potentially harmful to the fetus, as well as the mother. Weight reduction should be started after delivery.[57]

According to Hytten, the best reproductive performance in terms of perinatal mortality, preeclampsia and low birth weight babies is associated with the weight gain of healthy women "eating to appetite" as suggested by the 1 lb/week weight gain during the last month of gestation. Approximately eight pounds of weight gain is "maternal stores," fat stored mostly in subcutaneous deposits around the trunk and upper thighs. Early fat stores in pregnancy act as a buffer against possible deprivation in late pregnancy, when the fetus makes its greatest demands in growth.[34]

The increased nutritional requirements of pregnancy can be seen by reviewing the RDA chart (see Table 1–6). The specific cost of pregnancy is remarkably constant, although the components change. In early pregnancy, the increased calories of 300 kcal/day is for fat storage. In late pregnancy, the additional 300 kcal/day is almost entirely for maintenance needs. Protein, vitamin and mineral requirements are obviously increased to meet the demands of the growing fetus. The actual iron requirement for the fetus and to replace iron from blood lost by the mother at delivery amounts to approximately 500 mg. An additional peak requirement of 3–4 mg daily cannot be met by ordinary diets, and use of iron supplements is recommended.

It might be of greater meaning to interpret the RDAs for pregnant women by comparing them with an actual daily prenatal diet for an adult, healthy female. To ensure calcium and vitamin D requirements, one quart of milk or the equivalent in cheese or cottage cheese is recommended. To meet additional protein needs, meat servings should be increased to 3–4 oz twice daily. Five or more servings of fruit and vegetables assure the necessary vitamins and minerals if two servings are citrus (ascorbic acid) and one is a dark green or yellow vegetable (vitamin A). In addition to these caloric sources, bread and cereals and some form of fat should complete the diet to meet additional energy requirements.

Teenagers and poorly nourished persons should increase their intake, especially that of protein, to a total intake of 85 gm/day. The physician and dietitian must impress upon the patient the proper proportion of animal protein and exactly how much milk or its equivalent is needed. One cannot simply tell a patient to "follow a good diet" and "eat a lot of proteins and milk."[54]

Again and again, it has been emphasized that reduced nutritional intake has a depressing effect on physical development. Malnutrition during the period of rapid brain growth will lead to some neurologic impairment.[36] Low socioeconomic status has been associated with depressed fetal growth, increased perinatal mortality and morbidity and decreased mental development and is likely due to suboptimal calorie and protein nutrition during pregnancy. Physiologic and epidemiologic evidence suggests that energy (or calories) is the most common factor limiting fetal growth and that intervention to improve nutrition during the last few months of pregnancy may have possible benefits.[55]

In a study reported by Osofsky, more information was obtained about the quality of nutritional intake during pregnancy for women in an urban poverty setting and the relationship of nutrition to delivery and early infant development. Repeated nutritional assessments were made on 118 low income women who had registered at the hospital clinic prior to the 28th week of pregnancy. In addition, 122 comparable women provided with protein-mineral supplementation were studied. Demographic information, histories and physical examinations were obtained. Medical assessments were carried out throughout pregnancy, labor, delivery and postpartum. The infants were assessed medically and with Brazelton Neonatal Behavioral Assessment. Mothers who received protein-mineral supplements were less likely to develop preeclampsia and had fewer complications during labor and delivery, but no significant effect on infant development was observed.[49]

From this study, several hypotheses or suggestions were made. First, nutritional adequacy may be of benefit in the prevention of specific obstetrical problems, especially preeclampsia. Second, had there been significant evidence of deprivation, the infant medical and psychological measurements might have demonstrated greater abnormality. Third, *all* subjects received medical attention on *several* occasions, which promoted better medical health and more nutritious eating habits. Thus, perhaps good, continuous medical care might decrease the deleterious effects of undernutrition.[49]

Toxemia of pregnancy is not fully understood and its management is quite controversial. The Committee from the National Research Council found no evidence that excessive weight gain (fat or fluid) causes toxemia. As a matter of fact, women who are markedly underweight at conception show a higher incidence of toxemia. In addition, low income groups suffer a higher incidence of toxemia with an increased frequency of glomerular lesions. This is related to the degree of nutritional deprivation and associated hypoproteinemia.[57] It cannot be overemphasized that excessive weight gain or elevated blood pressure should not be equated with acute toxemia in all patients. Therefore, salt should not be grossly restricted unless the diagnosis of toxemia has been established. Retention of sodium is the *function* of toxemia; salt is *not* its cause.[48] Generally, management of the toxemic patient involves increasing water intake and enforcing complete bed rest. In true "toxemia," marked weight loss accompanies decreases in blood pressure to normal. For patients with edema, salt is restricted after the origin of the edema has been determined.

Nausea and vomiting are common problems in early pregnancy. Hormonal changes, as well as emotional factors, have been suggested as possible causes. Although dehydration, electrolyte and acid-base disturbances and starvation seldom become serious problems, some women may become gravely ill and require hospitalization for intravenous therapy. The usual therapy for patients who are not seriously ill is small, frequent feedings. Soda crackers often relieve nausea.

For women anticipating breast-feeding, further additions to the diet must be made to meet the even greater nutritional requirements. The requirements for lactating women can be found at the bottom of Table 1–6. The production of 850 ml of milk per day yields a loss of 600 kcal.[14] Six or more servings of fruits and vegetables with two servings of citrus and one serving of dark green or deep yellow vegetables are recommended to supply the higher amounts of ascorbic acid and vitamin A required.

Support for the nutritional needs during pregnancy are as follows:

1. There is a positive association between the weight gain of the mother and the birth weight of the infant.

2. A low protein intake has a role in the development of nutritional anemia, low birth weight infants, mental retardation, toxemias of pregnancy and suboptimal postnatal health of both infant and mother.

3. There is no scientific justification for prescribing vitamin-mineral supplements to pregnant women, with the possible exception of folic acid and iron. Vitamin and mineral supplements should not be substituted for adequate intake of nutrients.[22, 43]

Geriatric Nutrition

Eating should be a genuine pleasure at any age, and especially in old age, it should not be a chore or a dietary experiment. Alvarez has commented that older people think they need some special diet that is full of vitamins, certain proteins and "health foods." However, they need only a normal diet if they eat plenty of food of various types. Aging farmers rarely think of changing their diets "because they are getting old." Hippocrates supposedly said that the very fat person rarely reaches old age and that you need to keep your weight down "if you want to be healthy at 80."[1]

In Australia, most of the elderly seen at Hornsby and District Hospital appear to be consuming an adequate diet. Quite a few receive Meals-on-Wheels, which probably is an important factor in achieving adequate nutrition. Some of the aged are eating foods low in vitamin C, calcium, iron, possibly folic acid and vitamin B complex, which indicates that some changes in dietary habits are needed. If anemia is present, iron preparations are given, and the diet is revised.[17]

Surveys in the United Kingdom in 1967 and 1973 revealed little primary subnutrition due to lack of funds. Those with minimum incomes relied on cheaper but nutritional foods. Poverty occurred because of undue pride or ignorance of available financial help. Food fads and faulty dietary advice were more likely to lead to poor nutrition. Men over 75 years of age who lived alone were the most likely to have poor nutrition. Lack of dentures or poorly fitting dentures required soft food, making the diet very monotonous. Undernutrition usually had multiple causes, which included physical and mental illness or disability, loneliness, social isolation and bereavement. Relatives played an important role in caring for the elderly at home. Maintaining adequate nutrition was threatened by a drop in income at retirement and then later if people outlived their savings. It was suggested that there be courses in "preparation for retirement" and increased availability of lunch clubs and/or Meals-on Wheels.[18]

In America, some of the same problems were found. Lonely people do not prepare proper meals for themselves. Physical problems associated with degenerative diseases (arthritis, heart disease, incoordination) also complicate eating and meal preparation. From a study group of 3,500 elderly persons, one fourth ate less than three meals per day; one third ate no fruit; one fifth ate no vegetables; and one fifth consumed no milk or milk products.[51] As people reach 65 years of age, their diets are likely to be deficient in ascorbic acid, calcium and iron. In a survey in 1968, one fourth of the poor, older Americans said their food was tasteless. Many elderly people complained of lack of money, difficulty in preparing meals or securing food and need for dentures.[47]

According to Boykin, elderly persons bring with them a lifetime of food preferences, which should be considered on an individual basis when assessing nutritional status and developing a dietary plan. Nutritional adequacy or inadequacy is often the result of health status, including underlying physiologic and mental conditions. Foods that have deep significance or emotional meaning, such as "soul" foods, are influential in determining nutrient intake of older people, as well as those in other age groups. On occasion, an elderly person may eat these "soul" foods even if his "diet" does not permit them and risk the consequences. Therefore, health professionals must be cooperative in planning functional dietary regimens.[7]

In a study of the nutrition of 77 men and 187 women aged 65 and over and living at home in the United Kingdom, a seven-day dietary record was used to determine intakes of energy, protein, carbohydrate, sucrose, fat, vitamins and minerals. Mean intakes were less for women and (except for sucrose) fell slightly with age. The mean ener-

gy intake for men was 2,300 kcal/day; for women, 1,750 kcal/day. Men
derived more of their calories from bread, while women gained their
calories from cookies and cakes. Mean protein intake was 78 gm/day
for men and 60 gm/day for women. Protein provided about 15% of the
energy intake. Animal protein made up 54 gm/day for men and 43 gm/
day for women. Mean carbohydrate intake was 265 gm/day for men
and 194 gm/day for women. Sucrose intake averaged 76 gm/day for
men and 54 gm/day for women. Fat intake averaged 107 gm/day
for men and 86 gm/day for women. Of 31 subjects who met one or
more criteria for a low energy or protein intake, 15 were very overweight. Diagnosis of malnutrition was possible in 2% of the total
sample.[39] Calcium intake was below the national average, 900 mg/day
for men and 730 mg/day for women. The largest single source of calcium was milk, contributing only 33% of the intake for men and 44%
for women. Mean iron intake was greater in men (12.3 mg/day) than in
women (10 mg/day) and was marginally adequate. Potassium and
magnesium intakes were well below optimum levels: mean potassium
intake of 67 mEq/L per day for men and 55 mEq/L per day for women;
mean magnesium intake of 27 mEq/L per day in men and 19 mEq/L
per day in women.[40]

Malnutrition and disease in the aged has been depicted as a "vi-
cious cycle."

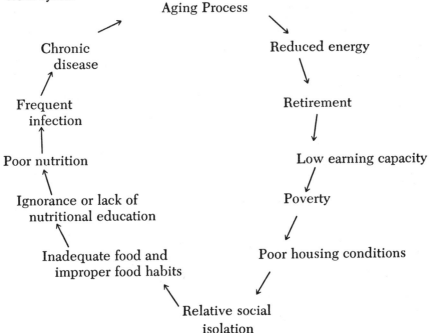

Glossitis in the elderly may be associated with niacin, folic acid, vitamin B_{12} or riboflavin deficiencies and can be associated with uremia or long- term systemic antibiotic therapy. Angular stomatitis can be associated with riboflavin, niacin or pyridoxine deficiencies or may be due to poorly fitting dentures.[41] The assessment of malnutrition in the aged must be done carefully and scrupulously, just as discussed earlier in the section on nutritional assessment.

Meals-on-Wheels has been a major factor in the solution of some of the problems of aging Americans. Providing one third to one half of the daily RDAs in the single delivered meal has been a boost in the right direction.

H. D. Kruse commented that the welfare state covers a person from the cradle to the grave, but nutrition exerts its influence from conception to the grave. Such an all-encompassing environmental factor is worthy of continual assessment and adjustment.

REFERENCES

1. Alvarez, W. C.: A normal diet and length of life, Geriatrics 26:81, 1971.
2. Beal, V. A.: Nutritional studies during pregnancy, II. Dietary intake, maternal weight gain, and size of infant, J. Am. Diet. Assoc. 58:321, 1971.
3. Bergman, S. G.: The atherosclerosis problem—pediatric and dietary aspects, Clin. Pediatr. 14:61, 1975.
4. Bistrian, B. R., et al.: Prevalence of malnutrition in general medical patients, J.A.M.A. 235:1567, 1976.
5. Blackburn, G. L., et al.: *Manual for Nutritional/Metabolic Assessment of the Hospitalized Patient* (Boston: New England Deaconess Hospital, Harvard Medical School, 1976).
6. Blumenthal, S., et al.: Risk factors for coronary artery disease in children of affected families, J. Pediatr. 87:1187, 1975.
7. Boykin, L. S.: Soul foods for some older Americans, J. Am. Geriatr. Soc. 23:380, 1975.
8. Bralove, M.: We're eating ourselves to death, Med. Times 100:255, 1972.
9. Breeling, J. L.: Adolescent nutrition, Ill. Med. J. 140:217, 1971.
10. Brubacher, G.: Biochemical studies for assessment of vitamin status in man, Bibl. Nutr. Dieta 20:31, 1974.
11. Butterworth, C. E.: The skeleton in the hospital closet, Nutr. Today 9:4, 1974.
12. Butterworth, C. E., and Blackburn, G. L.: Hospital malnutrition and how to assess the nutritional status of a patient, Nutr. Today 10:8, 1975.
13. Buzina, R.: Assessment of nutritional status and food composition surveys, Bibl. Nutr. Dieta 20:24, 1974.
14. Editorial: Calorie requirements of breast feeding, Br. Med. J. 3:721, 1970.
15. Clements, F. W.: Adolescent nutrition, Australas. Ann. Med. 19:377, 1970.
16. Clements, F. W.: Nutrition 1: What this series is about, Med. J. Aust. 1: 138, 1975.

17. Clements, F. W.: Nutrition of the elderly, Med. J. Aust. 1:473, 1975.
18. Cohen, C.: Social and economic factors in the nutrition of the elderly, Proc. Nutr. Soc. 33:51, 1974.
19. Committee on Nutrition, American Academy of Pediatrics: Childhood diet and coronary heart disease, Pediatrics 49:305, 1972.
20. Committee on Nutrition, American Academy of Pediatrics: Commentary on breast-feeding and infant formulas, including proposed standards for formulas, Pediatrics 57:278, 1976.
21. Committee on Nutrition, American Academy of Pediatrics: Salt intake and eating patterns of infants and children in relation to blood pressure, Pediatrics 53:115, 1974.
22. Cross, A. T., and Walsh, H. E.: Prenatal diet counseling, J. Reprod. Med. 7:265, 1971.
23. Dahl, L. K.: Salt and hypertension, Am. J. Clin. Nutr. 25:231, 1972.
24. Dahl, L. K.: Salt in processed baby foods, Am. J. Clin. Nutr. 21:787, 1968.
25. Darby, W. J.: Nutrition in the 1970s, Nutr. Rev. 30:31, 1972.
26. Davies, D. P.: Protein intake, osmolality, homeostasis and renal function in infancy, Postgrad. Med. J. 51 (suppl. 3):25, 1975.
27. Dugdale, A. E., Chen, S. T., and Hewitt, G.: Patterns of growth and nutrition in childhood, Am. J. Clin. Nutr. 23:1280, 1970.
28. Editorial: Clinical nutrition 1976: Where are we going? Ann. Intern. Med. 84:329, 1976.
29. Fomon, S. J.: *Infant Nutrition* (2d ed.; Philadelphia: W. B. Saunders Company, 1974).
30. Fomon, S. J.: What are infants fed in the United States? Pediatrics 56:350, 1975.
31. Garn, S. M., and Clark, D. C.: Nutrition, growth, development, and maturation: Findings from the ten-state nutrition survey of 1968–1970, Pediatrics 56:306, 1975.
32. Greaves, J. P., and Berry, W. T. C.: Medical, social and economic aspects of assessment of nutritional status, Bibl. Nutr. Dieta 20:1, 1974.
33. Guthrie, H. A.: Infant feeding practices—a predisposing factor in hypertension? Am. J. Clin. Nutr. 21:863, 1968.
34. Hytten, F. E.: Nutrition in pregnancy, Practitioner 212:459, 1974.
35. Isaksson, B.: Recommended methods used in the nutritional status assessment: Clinical signs and symptoms, Bibl. Nutr. Dieta 20:52, 1974.
36. Kallen, D. J.: Effects of nutrition on maternal-infant interaction, Fed. Proc. 34:1571, 1975.
37. Knittle, J. L., and Ginsberg-Fellner, F.: Can obesity be prevented? Pediatr. Ann. 4:28, 1975.
38. Lloyd, J. K.: Obesity in infancy, Postgrad. Med. J. 51 (suppl. 3):35, 1975.
39. Macleod, C. C., Judge, T. G., and Caird, F. I.: Nutrition of the elderly at home, I. Intakes of energy, protein, carbohydrates and fat, Age Ageing 3:158, 1974.
40. Macleod, C. C., Judge, T. G., and Caird, F. I.: Nutrition of the elderly at home, III. Intakes of minerals, Age Ageing 4:49, 1975.
41. Roa, D. B.: Malnutrition and disease in the aged, J. Am. Geriatr. Soc. 21:362, 1973.
42. Maslansky, E., et al.: Survey of infant feeding practices, Am. J. Public Health 64:780, 1974.

43. Maternal nutrition—what price? N. Engl. J. Med. 292:208, 1975.
44. Mongeau, E.: Nutrition in adolescence, Can. J. Public Health 62:330, 1971.
45. Naismith, D. J.: The dietary aetiology of accelerated growth in infancy, Postgrad. Med. J. 51 (suppl. 3):38, 1975.
46. Niswander, K. R.: Should pregnant patients gain more weight? Postgrad. Med. 48:133, 1970.
47. Nutrition and eating problems of the elderly, J. Am. Diet. Assoc. 58:43, 1971.
48. Nutrition and pregnancy. An invitational symposium, I, J. Reprod. Med. 7:199, 1971.
49. Osofsky, H. J.: Relationships between prenatal medical and nutritional measures, pregnancy outcome, and early infant development in an urban poverty setting, I. The role of nutritional intake, Am. J. Obstet. Gynecol. 123:682, 1975.
50. Pearson, P. B.: Nutrition perspectives in the seventies, Nutr. Rev. 30:31, 1972.
51. Pelcovits, J.: Nutrition to meet the human needs of older Americans, J. Am. Diet. Assoc. 60:297, 1972.
52. Purvis, G. A.: What nutrients do our infants really get? Nutr. Today 8:28, 1973.
53. Food and Nutrition Board/National Research Council: *Recommended Dietary Allowances* (8th rev. ed.; Washington, D.C.: National Academy of Sciences, 1974).
54. Ross, R. A.: Nutrition and pregnancy. An invitational symposium, II. Nutrition in maternal and perinatal morbidity and mortality in a rural state, J. Reprod. Med. 7:245, 1971.
55. Rush, D.: Maternal nutrition during pregnancy in industrialized societies, Am. J. Dis. Child. 129:430, 1975.
56. Salans, L. B., Cushman, S. W., and Weismann, R. E.: Adipose cell size and number in nonobese and obese patients, J. Clin. Invest. 52:929, 1973.
57. Shanholtz, M. I.: Maternal nutrition and the course of pregnancy, Va. Med. Mon. 93:381, 1971.
58. Talwar, P. P.: Developing indices of nutritional level from anthropometric measurements on women and young children, Am. J. Public Health 65:1170, 1975.
59. Editorial: The changing emphasis in nutrition, Med. J. Aust. 1:123, 1975.
60. Townley, R. R. W.: Food for the infant—the place of infant formula, Food Nutr. Notes & Rev. 28:77, 1971.
61. Wirths, W.: Evaluation of energy expenditure and nutritional status in dietary surveys, Bibl. Nutr. Dieta 20:77, 1974.

Chapter 2 / Nutrition and Diet Therapy in Obesity

"OBESITY IS PRESENT when the body is loaded with excessive fat."[15] Obesity is considered to be a major health concern in today's population, since it may lead to cardiovascular problems. Individuals who become obese as children are apt to remain obese as adults; they have more difficulty losing fat and maintaining weight loss.

Obesity usually is the result of excessive food intake or, more specifically, caloric intake that exceeds the energy needs of the individual. According to Goldrick, "Pathological obesity, i.e., people who exceed their ideal body weight by more than 20%, constitutes the bulk of patients who seek the help of a dietetic service." Goldrick goes on to say that "approximately 50% of these unfortunates lose an insignificant amount of weight, and only 5% achieve anything like a satisfactory weight loss." Many have psychological problems and cannot be helped by diet alone. The long-term maintenance of ideal body weight by previously obese individuals is discouraging.[15]

Levine and Seligmann suggest that a safe, quick method for losing pounds that have taken years to accumulate is nonexistent.[23] Adhering to a sensible diet doggedly and patiently, which probably means establishing and maintaining new eating habits, is the only way to keep weight down.

Fad Diets and Fallacies

Fad diets seem to promise a quick and easy way to reduce; some even promise the impossible: "Eat all you want and still lose weight." Most fad diets are dubious, unsafe and/or mislabeled: "Zen Macrobiotic Diet," "Mayo Diet" (categorically disclaimed by the Mayo Clinic), "Air Force Diet" (*not* from the Air Force), "Drinking Man's Diet," "Calories Don't Count Diet," "Hindu Guru Diet" and "Low Carbohydrate Diet." Many of these diets are high in protein and low in carbohydrates. However, when the diet is discontinued, fat returns.[23] The truth is any food can make you "fat" if you eat too much of it. Calories are calories! One gram of carbohydrate furnishes 4 kcal, as does 1 gm of protein; 1 gm of fat supplies approximately 9 kcal. Weight reflects the amount of calories consumed minus the amount of calories burned. Therefore, calories in excess of those needed for energy are stored as body fat.

In 1974, Solomon reviewed the history of fad diets.[35] In 1941, *Harpers Bazaar* promoted the "Grapefruit Diet," which consisted of eating half of a grapefruit before each meal. Actually, this had the effect of reducing the appetite so that not as much food was eaten during the meal. The "Steak and Tomato Diet," published by *The Saturday Evening Post* in 1942, provided meals consisting of only steak and a medium-sized tomato, with a tomato at bedtime, if still hungry. These diets supplied 800 and 700 kcal respectively. After originating in France, the "Egg and Orange Diet" hit the U.S. in 1950. This diet supplied 550 kcal through consumption of 3 eggs and 2½ oranges each day.

The 1960s saw a large variety of fad diets. The "No-Hunger Rice Diet" was promoted in *Coronet* in 1960 and was a takeoff on Dr. Walter Kempner's "Rice Diet," which was developed 30 years before. The diet furnished 950 kcal per day. In 1962, *Look* published the "Meat and Mushroom Diet," which provided 700 kcal/day and consisted of 9 oz of meat and 20 fresh mushrooms per day. The following year, the "Hot Dog Diet" was printed in *Look*. This 900-kcal diet consisted of 3 pure beef franks per day, each wrapped in a piece of bread, plus condiments and some vegetables. In 1964, *Vogue* printed two diets, the "Egg and Wine Diet" and the "Nibbling Diet." The "Egg and Wine Diet" provided 1,200 kcal in the form of 5 eggs per day plus a 24-oz bottle of wine, which caused serum cholesterol to rise and assaulted the liver. The "Nibbling Diet" provided six meals a day for a total of 1,000 kcal; later, in 1970, *McCall's* published the "Snack Diet," which was based on the same principle. Since most "fat" people eat only one meal each day, the "Nibbling" and "Snack" diets produced results by reducing the total amount of calories consumed.

Other diets proposed over the years include: "Vegetable and Fruit Diet," "Milk Diet," "Skim Milk and Banana Diet," "Strawberry and Cream Diet" and the "Pumpkin-Carrot Diet." Plato was the father of the vegetarian diet, which supposedly supplied 1,600 kcal. The "Milk Diet" originated a century ago and 20 years ago became the "Rockefeller Diet," which furnished 900 kcal in 4 liquid meals per day. The "Skim Milk and Banana Diet" originated in Pittsburgh's Highland Zoo area 35 years ago. This 625-kcal diet consisted of three 8-oz glasses of skim milk and a banana per day. The *Woman's Home Companion* printed the "Strawberry and Cream Diet," which supplied 550 kcal through 5 cups of strawberries topped with 8 tablespoons of sour cream per day. Australia's "Pumpkin-Carrot Diet" consists of

½ pumpkin and 10 carrots per day, which provides less than 600 kcal. However, after two weeks, the dieter's skin turns yellowish-orange because of carotenemia; women noted irregular periods and were concerned about pregnancy.[35]

In addition to being nutritionally unsound, these diets are monotonous, and most people tire of them quickly. Besides, weight lost quickly is usually regained when customary eating habits are resumed. Successful and consistent dieting requires effort and willpower. If an overweight person is serious about wanting excess pounds to dwindle, he must adhere to a sensible diet faithfully, be patient and hopeful and keep weight down by establishing and maintaining new eating habits that will continue for life.

Dieters hold many common fallacies:

"Since I've been dieting, my stomach has shrunk, and I don't have to eat so much."

"The best way to reduce is to skip lunch."

"Water is very fattening."

"Toasted bread has fewer calories than untoasted bread."

"Whole wheat or protein bread has fewer calories than white bread."

"Oleomargarine has a lower calorie content than butter."

"Exercise increases your appetite."

"Fruit juices are not fattening."

"Grapefruit can make you slimmer."

Formula and Chemically Defined Diets

"There is not enough known about nutrition to guarantee that formulas contain all the nutrients needed by the normal individual; this kind of dieting does not help the overweight person to learn the difference between good and bad eating habits, and people grow tired of formula diets." This statement expresses the view of the Council on Foods and Nutrition.

Chemically defined liquid diets have been used in studies on obese subjects. Baird and associates treated five obese patients for up to one year on chemically defined diets of 60–360 kcal containing appropriate L-amino acids (15 gm), carbohydrates (30–45 gm), vitamins and minerals.[2] These patients had few complaints of hunger and accepted the diets well. Nitrogen balance was maintained; serum electrolytes and uric acid were normal. Moderate ketosis was present, and mean weight loss was 4.1 lb (1.8 kg) per week. Clinical abnormalities observed were alopecia, a symptomatic normochronic anemia, postural hypotension and hypercholesterolemia. All these aberrations abated after patients resumed normal diets. Baird concluded that these particular chemically defined diets offered an acceptable and safer form of weight reduction than complete starvation for patients with severe or refractory obesity.

Ketogenic Diets

Low carbohydrate, ketogenic diets of various kinds have been promoted in cycles over the past 25 years as "effective" and "miraculous" approaches to weight reduction. These diets are not new or "revolutionary," since diets were devised nearly a century ago to eliminate sweet and starchy foods but permit meat as desired. All these diets have major features in common: (1) low to very low carbohydrate content; (2) no restriction in protein or fat; and (3) no limitations on calories. More recently, two physicians have lent their names to low carbohydrate diets, Dr. Stillman's *The Doctor's Quick Weight Loss Diet* and *Dr. Atkin's Diet Revolution: The High Calorie Way to Stay Thin Forever*. Although the proponents of these diets claim "universal and painless success," little if any decrease in obesity has been reported.[28]

The ketogenic diet recommended by Dr. Atkin restricted carbohydrate intake to less than 40 gm/day.[8] Dr. Stillman's diet is rich in protein and fat and is essentially carbohydrate-free. The diet proposed by Piscatelli and associates was outlined as follows: 800 – 1,000 kcal, 70% kcal as fat, 20% as protein and 10% as carbohydrates. This ketogenic diet offered no advantages in the amount of weight loss obtainable.[28] Unless a weight-reducing diet provides for a decrease in energy intake, it cannot be effective. Principally, weight loss on low carbohydrate, ketogenic diets is due to the consumption of fewer kcal.

Ketosis results from excessive mobilization of free fatty acids (FFA) stimulated by a deficiency of calorigenic substrates. If carbohydrate intake is limited, a concomitant decline in the supply of glucose results in diversion of any citric acid intermediates available in the liver to form glucose. The combination of increased FFA and diversion of citric acid cycle intermediates results in increased oxidation by the liver of FFA to D-3-oxybutyrates (Figure 2 – 1).

The limited intake from a high fat, adequate protein and low carbohydrate diet results in more severe ketosis than that produced by starvation. The primary difference is that the liver of the individual on a protein and fat diet is presented with a greater load of amino acids for metabolism than is that of the starved individual. The metabolism of

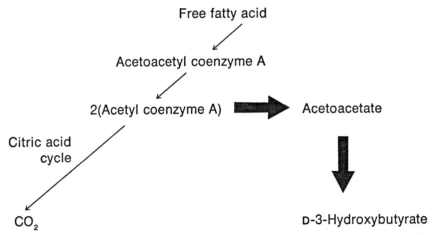

Fig 2–1.—Pathway responsible for the increased ketone formation resulting from calorie restriction.

amino acids involves later steps in the citric acid cycle and may thereby further reduce the capacity of this pathway to oxidize acetoacetyl coenzyme A arising from FFA and divert even more acetyl groups to form acetoacetate.

Ketogenesis may be looked upon as a mechanism that allows the liver to oxidize large quantities of FFA in a tightly coupled system of oxidative phosphorylation without increasing its total energy production. The complete oxidation of 1 M palmitate via the citric acid cycle produces 129 M adenosine triphosphate, whereas only 33 M are produced when acetoacetate is the end product.

The advantages of ketogenic diets are questionable. It has been suggested that ketones excreted in the urine are "wasted energy"; however, muscle and brain can utilize ketones, and caloric balance is affected minimally by urinary loss of ketones. Anorexia is produced by ketosis, but nausea can also result.

There are dangers associated with a diet low in carbohydrates and high in fat. Hyperlipidemia may be induced, and an increased risk of coronary heart disease is associated with hyperlipidemia. These diets may also cause an increase in serum uric acid concentration, because renal clearance of uric acid is inhibited by elevated serum ketones. An increase in serum uric acid concentration may exacerbate gout in patients with gouty diathesis. Other problems associated with low carbohydrate diets are postural hypotension and ketone accumulation producing an acidotic state.[7]

Starvation Diets

Prolonged fasting has been extensively studied as a means of weight reduction. The advantages of this approach to weight reduction are rapid weight loss achieved and the anorectic effect of the resulting ketosis. However, the ideal weight reducing program should produce fat mobilization without catabolism of lean body tissue, which is not the case in starvation. Several investigators have shown that during fasting one sees a markedly negative nitrogen balance. Benoit et al. reported that during a 10-day fast the mean weight loss was 9.6 kg, but 64.6% of this weight loss was due to loss of lean body tissue and was accompanied by a significant loss of intra- and extracellular water and electrolytes.[3] Bolinger and co-workers also showed that 40% of the weight loss during fasting is due to loss of intra- and extracellular water.[4] Lean body tissue, water and electrolyte losses can be reduced by adding to the diet as little as 40 gm of protein and 1,500 mg of sodium. The water and electrolyte deficits are quickly replenished on refeeding. This results in rapid weight gain and presents a psychological hazard to the obese patient. Total fasting cannot be recommended for weight reduction in most situations. However, in desperate situations, for example, a patient with morbid obesity who is in congestive heart failure, it may be a resort.

Surgical Treatment

In 1969, Payne and co-workers reported their opinion of the jejunoileal bypass in the treatment of obesity. They felt it was of definite benefit to patients whose obesity presented a hazard to health but not to patients who sought a 25–50-lb weight loss. The jejunocolic shunt should not be performed as the initial attempt to control obesity and should not be performed on patients with well-established cardiovascular disease. The physician and patient should have a relationship based on mutual respect, trust and responsibility, since cooperation is essential. This procedure should be considered as investigative and should not be undertaken unless facilities are available to handle complications.[26]

In 1970, Scott and Sandstead made a clinical and metabolic appraisal of the jejunoileal shunt in 11 carefully selected patients with gross obesity. Although early results were good in 7 of the 11 patients, specific nutritional deficits were found in the others and were cause for concern. Vitamins A and C and magnesium deficits were found in several patients, and fatty liver was seen in others. The investigators concluded that the jejunoileal shunt should be considered experimental in the treatment of morbid obesity and could not be recommended for wide therapeutic application at that time.[33]

The following year, Scott and Sandstead reported a new technique for intestinal bypass. The principle of this technique was to unite a very short segment of proximal jejunum to a very short segment of terminal ileum and maintain the important "braking" effect of the ileocecal valve in alimentary continuity, reducing the chyme in the bypassed jejunoileum by drainage into the transverse colon or sigmoid. Their experience with 12 obese patients indicated a satisfactory rate of weight loss in all but one, an associated reduction in serum lipids and a minimal problem with diarrhea.[32]

In 1973, Payne and his associates reported on their 16 years of experience with end-to-side intestinal bypass surgery for treatment of morbid obesity. They claimed satisfactory results and low morbidity in the majority of patients. "The mortality is acceptable considering the size of these patients and their numerous associated diseases." They were concerned with noted liver changes but felt these changes

TABLE 2-1.—COMPLICATIONS OF
JEJUNOILEAL BYPASS*

COMPLICATION	%
Hypokalemia	23
Hypocalcemia	22
Hypoalbuminemia	9
Metabolic acidosis	14
Elevated liver enzymes	41
Hyperbilirubinemia	6
Arthritis: Men	10
Women	19
Urinary calculi: Men	24
Women	10
Cholelithiasis: Men	10
Women	9
Liver impairments: Men	2
Women	6
Major emotional upset: Men	8
Women	9
Rehospitalization requirement: Men	49
Women	51
Deaths	8

*Study of 230 patients from DeWind, L. T., and Payne, J. H.: Intestinal bypass surgery for morbid obesity, J.A.M.A. 236:2298, 1976.

were reversible. Again, they reemphasized that bypass operation should be performed only on carefully selected patients.[27]

Table 2–1 outlines the results of a later study of 230 patients who underwent jejunoileal bypass surgery.

A case report by Mangla and co-workers described one of the serious complications that might result from jejunoileal bypass surgery. A 41-year-old white female who had been obese since adolescence had normal liver function tests except for mild elevation of alkaline phosphatase before surgery. Her liver appeared normal during the operation; so a biopsy was not done. However, for 25 months following surgery she progressed through fatty metamorphosis to cirrhosis and death. A poor diet had produced malnutrition and diarrhea, which contributed to her unwillingness to eat. With dietary control, liver function improved, but terminal failure of her ultimately cirrhotic liver prevented protein intake of any kind, and she died of hepatic failure and starvation.[24]

In 1974, Randolph and his associates reported results of intestinal bypass surgery for children and adolescents that appeared to parallel those observed in adults. They claimed these patients could deal with the operation and postoperative problems as well as adults. There was no apparent interference with skeletal growth after the bypass. The investigators recommended jejunoileal bypass surgery for adolescents and children with marked obesity who could not effectively reduce by diet alone.[29]

In summary, surgical approaches should be reserved for those patients with marked obesity in whom the traditional approaches of caloric restriction have failed.

CASE PRESENTATION.—V. L. is a 60-year-old white female who has been obese most of her life and has weighed as much as 355 pounds. In February, 1972, the patient and her son, who also was obese, were seen in the nutrition clinic. The patient was hypertensive, and her past medical history was noncontributory, except for previous hospitalizations for rheumatoid arthritis. The family history disclosed that her son and daughter also suffered from obesity and hypertension and that her husband had died from leukemia at the age of 62.

Physical examination revealed an overweight female with blood pressure 160/110 mm Hg, pulse 72 beats/min and regular, senile keratosis on forehead, clear chest and soft abdomen. Lab work showed complete blood count (CBC), urine aliquot (UA), blood urea nitrogen (BUN), creatinine and electrolytes within normal limits, as was serum cholesterol (168 mg/dl).

The patient was placed on a 1,000 kcal, 1,000 mg sodium diet and was followed by the nutrition clinic. Over a period of two years, the patient lost 190 lb. The patient's weights were as follows:

Dates	Weight (in lb)
4/11/72	291
10/15/72	222
1/01/73	202
7/11/73	169½
12/19/73	177
5/01/74	165
1/02/75	210
1/10/75	208¾

The patient began gaining weight after not adhering to the diet. She was given more encouragement to continue with her diet and told to return to the Nutrition Clinic for follow-up.

CASE PRESENTATION.—G. L. is a 27-year-old white male son of V. L. He developed hypertension in high school and took 25 mg guanethidine hydrochlorothiazide daily. The patient lost approximately 200 lb between high school and age 24.

In February, 1972, the patient was seen in the nutrition clinic with complaints of dizziness on rising for the previous four months without nausea, sweating and palpitations. He complained of cold intolerance; dry, flaky, scaly skin; dry, fine hair with loss at each combing; decreased bowel movements from 2 to 3 per day to one every 1 to 2 days; voice change (lower); and mild weakness for four months.

His past medical history was noncontributory, except for two previous hospitalizations for hypertension in 1967 and 1970. The family history disclosed that his mother and sister suffered from obesity and hypertension and that his father had died from leukemia at age 62.

Physical examination revealed an overweight young man with blood pressure 110/70 mm Hg, pulse 50 beats/min and regular, dry and flaky skin, clear chest and soft abdomen with questionable liver edge. Lab work showed 7.7 μg/dl true thyroxine; 5.1 μg/dl plasma cortisol, 17 ketosteroids and normal 6-hour glucose tolerance test. CBC, UA, BUN, creatinine, thyroid antibodies and electrolytes were within normal limits.

The patient was placed on a 1,000 kcal diet and was followed by the nutrition clinic. The patient's weights were as follows:

Dates	Weight (in lb)
2/22/72	218
5/12/72	189
7/18/72	172
12/24/73	200
4/25/74	198
9/19/74	210
2/01/75	234½
2/15/75	222½
2/22/75	219½

The patient's weight began fluctuating in 1973 and 1974. In February 1975, he resumed dieting and follow-up by the nutrition clinic.

TABLE 2-2.—SUGGESTED WEIGHTS FOR HEIGHTS AND BASAL METABOLIC RATES (BMR) OF ADULTS°

		MEN			WOMEN		
HEIGHT		MEDIAN WEIGHT		BMR	MEDIAN WEIGHT		BMR
(IN)	(CM)	(LB)	(KG)	(KCAL/DAY)	(LB)	(KG)	(KCAL/DAY)
60	152				109 ± 9	50 ± 4	1,399
62	158				115 ± 9	52 ± 4	1,429
64	163	133 ± 11	60 ± 5	1,630	122 ± 10	56 ± 5	1,487
66	168	142 ± 12	64 ± 5	1,690	129 ± 10	59 ± 5	1,530
68	173	151 ± 14	69 ± 6	1,775	136 ± 10	62 ± 5	1,572
70	178	159 ± 14	72 ± 6	1,815	144 ± 11	66 ± 5	1,626
72	183	167 ± 15	76 ± 7	1,870	152 ± 12	69 ± 5	1,666
74	188	175 ± 15	80 ± 7	1,933			
76	193	182 ± 16	83 ± 7	1,983			

°From Food and Nutrition Board, National Research Council: *Recommended Dietary Allowances* (8th rev. ed.; Washington, D.C.: National Academy of Sciences, 1974).

Determining "Ideal" Weight

There are several ways of determining a patient's "ideal" body weight, but most physicians rely on various height/weight tables. The most frequently used table is that published by the Metropolitan Life Insurance Company. However, a more accurate table of suggested weight for height is presented in the *Recommended Dietary Allowances*, published by the National Research Council. Table 2–2 shows suggested weights for heights of adults in the 1974 edition.

A simple rule for estimating desirable weight for adults is as follows:

1. For women, allow 100 lb for the first 5 feet and 5 lb for each additional inch;

2. For men, allow 110 lb for the first 5 feet and 5 lb for each additional inch; and

3. Allow 10% variation above or below the calculated weight for individual differences.

Determining Kilocalorie Levels

Determining the appropriate kcal level for a given individual depends upon several considerations, such as age, activity level and basal metabolic rate. However, one may often want to make a rapid calculation of an individual's kcal requirement. Multiplying the desirable weight in lb by 18 for a woman is approximately equal to the number of kcal required for moderate activity. For a man, multiplying the desirable weight in lb by 21 is approximately equal to the number of kcal required for moderate activity.

Kilocalories required for specific activities may be determined from charts, such as the one in Table 2–3.

Another means of determining kcal levels was adapted by the Food and Nutrition Board of the National Academy of Sciences. This method is based on energy expenditure and adjustment of kcal allowances for adults. Explanations of various activity levels are given in the RDAs. Kilocalorie allowances should be adjusted for the adult according to age. Energy requirements decline progressively after early adulthood because physical activity is curtailed, and the resting metabolic rate declines. Decline of resting metabolism is 2% per decade in adults. For persons over 50 years of age, energy allowances should be reduced to 90% of the amount required for mature adults.

For weight loss, Williams recommends the following kcal adjustment: To lose 1 lb/week, subtract 500 kcal daily; to lose 2 lb/week, subtract 1,000 kcal daily. Two pounds per week is the most practical weight loss. This estimation is based on: 1 lb of body fat equals 454

TABLE 2–3.—ENERGY COST OF ACTIVITIES EXCLUSIVE OF BASAL METABOLISM AND INFLUENCE OF FOOD*

ACTIVITY	KCAL/KG/HR	ACTIVITY	KCAL/KG/HR
Bicycling (century run)	7.6	Organ playing (30% to 40% of energy hand work)	1.5
Bicycling (moderate speed)	2.5	Painting furniture	1.5
Bookbinding	0.8	Paring potatoes	0.6
Boxing	11.4	Playing ping pong	4.4
Carpentry (heavy)	2.3	Piano playing (Mendelssohn's songs)	0.8
Cello playing	1.3		
Crocheting	0.4	Piano playing (Beethoven's Appassionata)	1.4
Dancing (foxtrot)	3.8		
Dishwashing	1.0	Piano playing (Liszt's Tarantella)	2.0
Dressing and undressing	0.7	Reading aloud	0.4
Driving automobile	0.9	Running	7.0
Eating	0.4	Sawing wood	5.7
Fencing	7.3	Sewing (hand)	0.4
Horseback riding (walk)	1.4	Sewing (foot-driven machine)	0.6
Horseback riding (trot)	4.3	Sewing (motor-driven machine)	0.4
Horseback riding (gallop)	6.7	Shoemaking	1.0
Ironing (5-lb iron)	1.0	Singing (in loud voice)	0.8
Knitting sweater	0.7	Sitting quietly	0.4
Laundry (light)	1.3	Skating	3.5
Lying still (awake)	0.1		

*From Krause, M. V., and Hunscher, M. S.[21]

gm; 1 gm of *body fat* equals 7.7 kcal; 454 gm multiplied by 7.7 kcal/gm is equal to 3,496 kcal/lb body fat, which is nearly 3,500 kcal. If 3,500 kcal is divided by 7 days, the result is 500 kcal/day, the amount of kcal that must be subtracted daily for a 1 lb/week weight loss.[38]

General Aspects and Controversy of Dietary Management in Obesity

Although weight reduction is a preventive measure that improves the exercise capacity of patients with chronic obesity and the body oxygen uptake, blood volume, cardiac output and arteriovenous difference,[1] controversy over how to manage the obese still exists. One of the controversies concerns meal frequency and "time factors." Finkelstein and Fryer demonstrated that meal frequency was not significant; it did not affect weight loss, nitrogen balance or total serum lipids and cholesterol.[11] However, Sassoon's review emphasized the time factors involved in convertibility of kcal to body fat.[30] In a study by Young and associates, oral glucose tolerance was reduced with one meal per day, but increased frequency of meals did not affect these results. Serum cholesterol and triglycerides were higher with one meal per day than with 3 or 6 meals per day.[39]

Another controversy, which was alluded to previously, is the composition of the weight reduction diet in terms of carbohydrate, protein and fat. Schauf's objective to lessen insulin secretion was accomplished by increasing intake of protein and certain fat-containing calories and by decreasing the intake of carbohydrate.[31] However, Bray saw no long-term differences in quantity of weight lost due to isocaloric substitutions of carbohydrate, protein or fat.[5] Grey and Kipnis concluded that the hyperinsulinemia characteristic of obesity may be a result, in part, of dietary factors rather than an exclusive consequence of insulin antagonism. Plasma insulin levels decreased 50% in patients on a low carbohydrate diet and increased on a high carbohydrate diet.[17]

Then, there is the question of when obesity began, the state of the fat cells in the body and what can be done for certain obese individuals. According to Burch, the number of fat cells reflects the state of nutrition during early periods of postnatal life. The size of the cells reflects the quantity "stuffed" into each fat cell after growth and cell proliferation cease.[7] According to Goldrick, the capacity of humans to accumulate fat is unlimited.[15] Obesity is a reflection of a general "maladaptation to the excess of food and labour saving appliances" of our culture. Reduction in food intake and more exercise are the keys to maintenance of ideal body weight.

In treating the obese adolescent, Hammar and others have made several suggestions: Help the patient feel more acceptable; help him make a more satisfactory adjustment to his life situation; and provide him with good nutritional education.[18]

In brief, suggestions for treating the obese adolescent are the same as those for the obese adult. Providing emotional support and encouragement, as well as good nutrition education, are just as important as establishing a "diet" per se for the overweight individual if he is to be successful with weight loss and maintenance.

REFERENCES

1. Alexander, J. K., and Peterson, K. L.: Cardiovascular effects of weight reduction, Circulation 45:310, 1972.
2. Baird, I. M., et al.: Clinical and metabolic studies of chemically defined diets in the management of obesity, Metabolism 23:645, 1974.
3. Benoit, F. L., Martin, R. L., and Watten, R. H.: Changes in body composition during weight reduction in obesity: Balance studies comparing effects of fasting and a ketogenic diet, Ann. Intern. Med. 63:604, 1965.
4. Bolinger, R. E., et al.: Metabolic balance of obese subjects during fasting, Arch. Intern. Med. 118:3, 1966.
5. Bray, G. A., and Campfield, L. A.: Metabolic factors in the control of energy stores, Metabolism 24:99, 1975.
6. Brook, C. G., et al.: Adipose cell size and glucose tolerance in obese children and effects of diet, Arch. Dis. Child 48:301, 1973.
7. Burch, G. E.: Fat cells, nutrition and obesity, Am. Heart J. 82:839, 1971.
8. Council on Foods and Nutrition: A critique of low-carbohydrate ketogenic weight reduction regimens—a review of Dr. Atkin's diet revolution, J.A.M.A. 224:1415, 1973.
9. Davidson, M. D.: Effect of obesity on insulin sensitivity of human adipose tissue, Diabetes 21:6, 1972.
10. Drenick, E. J.: Starvation in the management of obesity, in Wilson, N. (ed.): *Obesity* (Philadelphia: F. A. Davis Company, 1969), pp. 191–203.
11. Finkelstein, B., and Fryer, B. A.: Meal frequency and weight reduction of young women, Am. J. Clin. Nutr. 24:465, 1971.
12. Garrow, J. S.: Diet and obesity, Proc. R. Soc. Med. 66:642, 1973.
13. Gastineau, C. F.: The prediction of weight loss on a reducing diet, Minn. Med. 43:255, 1960.
14. Goldman, J. K., et al.: Food intake in hypothalamic obesity, Am. J. Physiol. 227:88, 1974.
15. Goldrick, R. B.: Over nutrition—obesity, Food Nutr. Notes Rev. 28:87, 1971.
16. Goodhart, R. S., and Shils, M. E.: *Modern Nutrition in Health and Disease, Dietotherapy* (5th ed.; Philadelphia: Lea & Febiger, 1973).
17. Grey, N., and Kipnis, D. M.: Effect of diet composition on the hyperinsulinemia of obesity, N. Engl. J. Med. 285:827, 1971.

18. Hammar, S. L., Campbell, V., and Woolley, J.: Treating adolescent obesity: Long-range evaluation of previous therapy, Clin. Pediatr. 10:46 1971.
19. Johnson, H. L., et al.: Metabolic aspects of caloric restriction: Nutrient balances with 500 kilocalorie intakes, Am. J. Clin. Nutr. 24:913, 1971.
20. Kaufmann, N. A., et al.: Teenagers dieting for weight control, Nutr. Metab. 16:30, 1974.
21. Krause, M. V., and Hunscher, M. S.: *Food Nutrition and Diet Therapy* (5th ed.; Philadelphia: W. B. Saunders Company, 1972), p. 36.
22. Krzywicki, H. J., et al.: Metabolic aspects of caloric restriction (420 kilocalorie): Body composition changes, Am. J. Clin. Nutr. 25:67, 1972.
23. Levine, M. I., and Seligmann, J. H.: *Your Overweight Child* (Cleveland: World Publishing Company, 1970).
24. Mangla, J. C., Hoy, W., Kim, Y., et al.: Cirrhosis and death after jejunoileal shunt for obesity, Am. J. Dig. Dis. 19:759, 1974.
25. Mayer, J.: *Overweight, Causes, Cost and Control* (Englewood Cliffs, N. J.: Prentice-Hall, Incorporated, 1968).
26. Payne, J. H., and De Wind, L. T.: Surgical treatment of obesity, Am. J. Surg. 118: 141,1969.
27. Payne, J. H., et al.: Surgical treatment of morbid obesity: Sixteen years of experience, Arch. Surg. 106:432, 1973.
28. Piscatelli, R. L., Cerchio, G. M., and Kleit, S. A.: The ketogenic diet in the management of obesity, in Wilson, N. (ed.): *Obesity* (Philadelphia: F. A. Davis Company, 1969), p. 185.
29. Randolph, J. G., Weintraub, W. H., and Riggs, A.: Jejunoileal bypass for morbid obesity in adolescents, J. Pediatr. Surg. 9:341, 1974.
30. Sassoon, H. F.: Time factors in obesity, Am. J. Clin. Nutr. 26:776, 1973.
31. Schauf, G. E.: Diet and management of obesity: and Bray, G.A.: Reply to Dr. Schauf, Am. J. Clin. Nutr. 24:387, 1971.
32. Scott, H. W., et al.: Experience with a new technique of intestinal bypass in the treatment of morbid obesity, Ann. Surg. 174:560, 1971.
33. Scott, H. W., et al.: Jejunoileal shunt in the treatment of morbid obesity, Ann. Surg. 171:770, 1970.
34. Sohar, E., and Sneh, E.: Followup of obese patients: 14 years after a successful reducing diet, Am. J. Clin. Nutr. 26:845, 1973.
35. Solomon, N.: Improper dieting—a health hazard, Md. State Med. J. 23:42, 23:61, 23:70, 1970.
36. Stunkard, A. J., and Rush, J.: Dieting and depression reexamined—a critical review of reports of untoward responses during weight reduction for obesity, Ann. Intern. Med. 81:526, 1974.
37. Tullis, I. F.: Rational diet construction for mild and grand obesity, J.A.M.A. 226:70, 1973.
38. Williams, S. R.: *Nutrition and Diet Therapy* (St. Louis: C. V. Mosby Company, 1969).
39. Young, C. M., et al.: Frequency of feeding, weight reduction and nutrient utilization, J. Am. Diet. Assoc. 59:473, 1971.

Chapter 3 / Nutrition in Diseases of the Gastrointestinal Tract

MUCH OF THE nutritional therapy for diseases of the gastrointestinal tract has been based on supposition. For many years, the diet for patients with peptic ulcers has been composed of "bland" foods, which supposedly stimulate less secretion and do not physically irritate the ulcer. After much investigation, the bland diet was found to be no more efficacious than a regular diet that excluded beverages containing alcohol or caffeine. In addition, diseases such as diverticular disease of the colon, ulcerative colitis and regional enteritis were once treated with low residue diets, but perhaps should be treated with a high residue diet, since no beneficial effect has resulted from low residue diets. With diverticular disease, low residue diets seem to produce isolated segments of high pressure and complete contraction of the colon, which increases the problem for patients.[40] There are similar reversals of opinion in the dietary management of diseases of the liver and gallbladder, since many diets are still quite controversial.

It is the purpose of this chapter to review the dietary management (both old and new) of certain abnormal conditions of the gastrointestinal tract. It will be your decision as to how you would "dietarily" treat patients with these conditions based on the material presented, your own personal prejudices and, most of all, the tolerances of your patients. The key to diet therapy for gastrointestinal diseases is individualization. It is not our purpose to undertake a complete review of gastrointestinal physiology. We simply will review those elements of the digestive process which are pertinent to the discussion of the nutritional management of gastrointestinal disease.

Physiology of the Stomach and Small Intestine

Stomach

The stomach actually has three main functions: receiving food, retaining it during chemical digestion and slowly and intermittently passing liquid chyme to the duodenum and small intestine. Receiving food is an uncomplicated process unless the esophagus or cardiac sphincter is diseased or damaged in some way. However, the process of digestion is more complex. Hormones, enzymes and other secretions of the stomach will be reviewed briefly.

41

At the thought, smell, or taste of food, the vagus nerve is triggered. It, in turn, stimulates the antrum of the stomach to produce the hormone gastrin. Distention of the stomach by food and exposure of the mucosa to products of protein digestion also may stimulate gastrin production. Gastrin then stimulates gastric secretion. Gastric secretions may be increased when the stomach receives certain anti-inflammatory agents (such as salicylates and glucocorticoids), caffeine and alcohol.

Gastric secretion is composed of water, inorganic ions, enzymes and their precursors, mucins, the intrinsic factor of Castle and many other substances in small amounts. Goblet cells produce mucous products (mucoproteins), composed of mucopolysaccharide and protein; mucus covers the mucosal lining to protect gastric mucosa against chemical, mechanical and thermal irritation.

Actually, the motor function of the stomach, that of passing chyme into the small intestine, is the most important, and it is not fully understood. Peristaltic activity starts shortly after ingested food increases the volume of the stomach. Contractions are limited to the pyloric region at first and then are followed by waves that begin higher in the fundus of the stomach. The rate of emptying is influenced by tonicity, consistency of foods, size of meals, composition of foods, presence of pain, emotional state and gastric disease, as well as other physiologic states.

Small Intestine

CARBOHYDRATES. — The principal locations for the digestion of carbohydrates are the mouth, the lumen of the small intestine and the brush border of the epithelial cells of the intestinal mucosa. In the mouth, alpha amylase acts on starch to break the alpha-D-glycosidic bonds producing maltose-D-glucose and smaller units of the starch molecule called starch dextrins. At this stage, starch has been reduced in size to an average chain of less than eight glucose units. The high level of acidity in the stomach stops the action of alpha amylase; therefore, little hydrolysis of carbohydrates occurs in the stomach. As the material enters the small intestine, the pH becomes alkalinzed by secretion of bile and pancreatic juices. The digestion of starch dextrins is continued by action of the pancreatic alpha amylase to form maltose, isomaltose and D-glucose. At this point, the intestinal lumen also contains dietary lactose and sucrose. Ingested cellulose is a polysaccharide with 1,4-β-D-glycosidic linkages, for which man has no hydrolytic enzyme; therefore cellulose is nondigestible. Disaccharides are hydrolyzed at the brush border by specific disaccharidases that are contained in the cell membrane. The resulting monosaccharides and glucose in the lumen pass into the portal blood system through which they are transported to the liver.

The absorption of sugars from the intestine is quite complex. Pentoses appear to cross the intestinal barrier by simple passive diffusion. Other sugars, that is, D-glucose, D-fructose, D-galactose and possibly D-mannose, can be transported against a concentration gradient. This transport requires the transport of sodium. This process occurs primarily in the upper jejunum.

PROTEIN.—Dietary proteins are digested into their constituent amino acids by proteolytic enzymes and peptidases contained within the gastrointestinal tract. All proteolytic enzymes, except the intestinal peptidases, exist as zymogens, that is, larger protein precursors that must be converted to smaller molecules to be active. The hormone gastrin, which is secreted from the distal end of the stomach, stimulates the chief cells to release the zymogen pepsinogen. Pepsinogen is activated autocatalytically by the low pH of stomach contents. Under these acid conditions, the small amount of pepsinogen is cleaved to pepsin. The duodenum secretes the hormone secretin, which stimulates the pancreas to release its digestive juices. Secretion of both gastrin and secretin is stimulated by gastric distention and entry of chyme into the duodenum. Pancreatic juice in the duodenum contains the zymogens chymotrypsinogen, trypsinogen and procarboxypeptidase. The cascade of activation of these enzymes is illustrated in Figure

Fig 3–1.—Activation of zymogens.

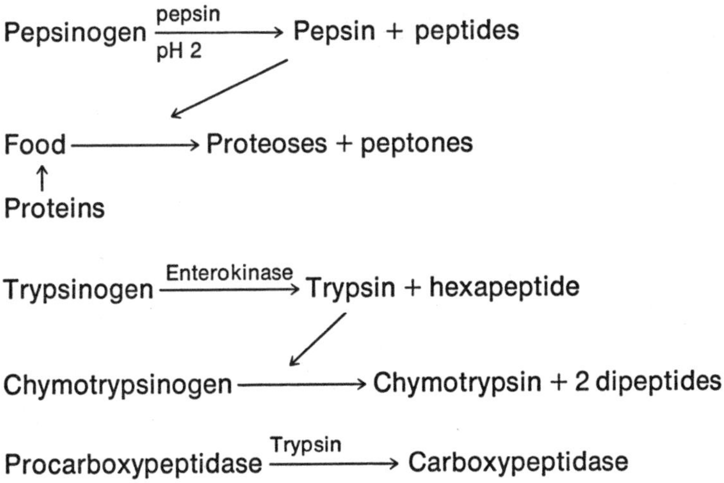

$$\text{Pepsinogen} \xrightarrow[\text{pH 2}]{\text{pepsin}} \text{Pepsin + peptides}$$

$$\text{Food} \longrightarrow \text{Proteoses + peptones}$$

$$\uparrow$$
Proteins

$$\text{Trypsinogen} \xrightarrow{\text{Enterokinase}} \text{Trypsin + hexapeptide}$$

$$\text{Chymotrypsinogen} \longrightarrow \text{Chymotrypsin + 2 dipeptides}$$

$$\text{Procarboxypeptidase} \xrightarrow{\text{Trypsin}} \text{Carboxypeptidase}$$

3-1. Proteolytic enzymes are specific for cleaving protein chains at certain amino acid residues. The products of these cleavages are free amino acids, dipeptides and small peptides. The small peptides are further hydrolyzed in the intestinal mucosal cells by aminopeptidase and dipeptidases.

LIPID.—Dietary lipid is composed of triglyceride, small amounts of phosphoglycerides, cholesterol esters and cholesterol. These lipids must be emulsified, digested by hydrolytic enzymes and absorbed into the intestinal mucosal cells. Emulsification of the lipids occurs in the duodenum, where lipids interact with bile. The purpose of emulsification is to transform the poorly soluble dietary lipids into mixed micelles, which are aggregates formed in aqueous solution by a substance composed of both polar and nonpolar components. Nonpolar components orient themselves inside the aggregate, while polar groups interact with the surrounding water molecules on the outside. This renders them miscible in water. In this form, lipids can be acted upon by digestive enzymes and become hydrolyzed. Three hydrolytic enzymes—pancreatic lipase, cholesterol esterase and phospholipase-A—are produced by the pancreas and are secreted into the duodenum. Pancreatic lipase catalyzes the partial hydrolysis of triglyceride-containing, long-chain fatty acids. Digestion of triglyceride usually stops at the 2-monoglyceride. Both the 2-monoglyceride and fatty acid can pass through the cell membrane and are diffused into the mucosal cells of the jejunum and ileum. Most of the dietary cholesterol is unesterified, but any cholesterol ester that is present is emulsified and hydrolyzed by the pancreatic cholesterol esterase to form cholesterol and fatty acids. The released cholesterol and fatty acids then diffuse from the micelles to the intestinal cell membranes. Absorption from other mixed micelles occurs by a similar passive process. The intestinal mucosal cells resynthesize the absorbed fatty acid and 2-monoglycerides into triglycerides. The lipid that is accumulated in the mucosal cell is then released into the lymph in the form of two micellar lipoproteins—chylomicrons and very low density lipoprotein. The lipoproteins then pass into the venous blood. The serum triglycerides are removed through the action of a hydrolytic enzyme, lipoprotein lipase, and the released fatty acids are taken up by the tissue. In contrast to long-chain fatty acids occurring in triglycerides, medium-chain triglycerides (MCT) can be absorbed intact. They pass directly into the portal vein as fatty acids and do not require micelle formation or esterification.

Nutrition in Diseases of the Stomach

Hiatal Hernia

One of the more common conditions affecting the upper gastrointestinal tract is herniation of part of the stomach through the diaphragmatic hiatus. Herniation is considered one of the most important mechanical gastrointestinal diseases but causes illness in only a small number of the people it affects. Heartburn or pyrosis is the most common complaint of these patients; other complaints are regurgitation, dysphagia, substernal or xyphoid pain and bleeding.[22]

Generally, medical management of herniation involves prevention of constipation and straining at the stool, weight reduction for obese patients, elevation of the head of the bed for semirecumbent sleeping and a diet of soft foods in small, frequent feedings. If regurgitation is frequent, then relatively bland foods are suggested, and highly seasoned or spicy foods are eliminated. Also, the patient is instructed to avoid reclining or engaging in strenuous physical activity after meals. It may also be necessary to stress the importance of eating slowly and chewing food well before swallowing. Often, patients with a hiatal hernia "eat on the run" and are keeping a "fast pace" in life. Sometimes, they eat only one large meal each day and thereby overdistend their stomachs once a day.

Any condition leading to recurrent vomiting or increased intra-abdominal pressure may worsen the problem of hiatal hernia and may result in further complications. Therefore, chronic cough should be treated vigorously, and tight belts or supports should be avoided. Complications of esophagitis or peptic ulcer must be treated with antacids and a diet that eliminates highly seasoned or spicy foods.

Gastritis

Gastritis is generally defined as an inflammation of the gastric wall, especially of the gastric mucosa, and is a fairly common disorder. It may be acute or chronic in nature. Acute gastritis may be divided into four types: (1) simple exogenous, (2) corrosive, (3) infectious (hematogenous) and (4) phlegmonous. Acute infectious gastritis, which is most common, arises from toxins or bacteria entering the stomach from the bloodstream. A diet avoiding known gastric irritants should be instituted if the patient can tolerate oral intake. Otherwise, intravenous feedings should be used to prevent dehydration and starvation.

Chronic nonspecific gastritis presents more of a problem clinically and can be divided into three types: (1) superficial, (2) atrophic and (3) hypertrophic. The etiology and pathogenesis of chronic gastritis is unknown. Infections, dietary indiscretions, alcohol, coffee, tobacco and nutritional deficiencies have been implicated; however, the evidence is inconclusive. Atrophic gastritis is more frequent with a gastric ulcer, whereas hypertrophic gastritis is more common with a duodenal ulcer. Atrophy of the gastric mucosa also occurs with pernicious anemia and gastric polyposis and sometimes with sprue, pellagra and iron deficiency anemia. A possible immune mechanism has been suggested as the cause of chronic gastritis.[22]

The course of disease in patients with chronic gastritis is persistent or recurrent, but the type, severity and distribution is unpredictable, even in the same individual. Vitamin B_{12} deficiency may develop in elderly women, but it rarely progresses to pernicious anemia. The associated weakness, loss of memory, mental depression, paresthesias and abdominal discomfort with flatulence frequently improve with vitamin B_{12} therapy. When atrophic gastritis is associated with an iron or vitamin deficiency, loss of appetite, fullness, vague epigastric pain, belching, nausea and vomiting are frequent complaints. These symptoms may be relieved by a "bland" diet, antispasmodic drugs and vitamin supplements.[22] Generally, individual patients learn the specific foods and seasonings that cause distress.

Peptic Ulcer

The mucosa of the normal stomach is protected by the mucosal barrier, which consists of the layer of mucous that lines the luminal surface of the epithelial cells and the mucosal cells that comprise the epithelial membrane. Hydrogen (H^+) ions, acetylsalicylic acid, bile salts and alcohol readily traverse the mucus layer to disrupt the barrier. The normal stomach is almost impermeable to a solution with pH 1.0 in the lumen. When the barrier is disrupted, however, hydrogen ions enter the mucosa in great quantities, and large amounts of pepsin are released. Back-diffusion of H^+ also stimulates release of histamine, which, in turn, increases H^+ secretion by parietal cells, increased capillary permeability and edema.

There is evidence to indicate that patients with a gastric ulcer have greater reflux of bile salts from the duodenum into the stomach than normal subjects. The greater reflux of bile salts, along with other sequences of events that result in release of histamine and vasodilatation, may contribute to increased bleeding after ingestion of aspirin. Aspirin also breaks the mucosal barrier. The pyloric sphincter in patients with a gastric ulcer does not contract normally in response to secretin or cholecystokinin, even after the ulcer has healed. However, pyloric malfunction is not the only answer.[30, 31]

According to Isenberg, peptic ulcer disease occurs in approximately 10% of the population of the United States, and the incidence of duodenal ulcers is about ten times greater than that of gastric ulcers. Ulcer disease is more prevalent in smokers than nonsmokers, and it is about three times more common in relatives of affected individuals than in the general population. Gastric ulcers may be due to increased duodenogastric reflux; duodenal ulcers may be caused by a nicotine-induced decrease in pancreatic bicarbonate secretion, which allows a lower duodenal pH. Persons with type O blood and who do not secrete blood group substances have a 2½ times greater incidence of ulcers than those with types A, B or AB blood and who secrete blood group substances.[30, 31]

Even though socioeconomic differences do not appear to affect the incidence of duodenal ulcer, gastric ulcer is seen a little more frequently in patients of lower socioeconomic classes. Drugs are often associated with the incidence of gastric ulcer, but aspirin is the only commonly used agent that may play an etiologic role. Evidence implicating corticosteroids, reserpine, phenylbutazone and indomethacin is inconclusive because few well-controlled studies have been conducted. Although investigators have claimed that ulcers are more prevalent in patients with chronic obstructive pulmonary disease, cirrhosis (with and without portacaval shunt), rheumatoid arthritis and hyperthyroidism, most studies have lacked satisfactory control populations; therefore, definite conclusions cannot be drawn.[22, 30, 31]

There is greater secretion of gastric acid and pepsin at rest and in response to gastric stimulation in patients with duodenal ulcer than in normal subjects. Increased sensitivity to gastric acid stimulants, increased secretory capacity and decreased inhibition of acid secretion may contribute to ulcer formation. Gastrin release is accentuated, and inhibition of gastrin-stimulated acid secretion is diminished at pH 2.5. Though ideas have been postulated, reasons for the physiologic defects are unknown; much more controlled research is necessary.[30, 31]

Therapeutic methods that affect healing and control of pain, recurrence and complications in patients with ulcers remain controversial. Antacids and anticholinergics are the primary therapeutic agents in ulcer management, while diet, sedation and tranquilizers have no demonstrated value. The discontinuance of smoking, hospitalization and limitation of aspirin ingestion expedite healing of gastric ulcers.[30, 31, 33]

Controversy regarding physiologic gastric rest through dietary con-

trol began during the nineteenth century. The Sippy regimen of inter-
spersing antacids with milk each hour was popular in that era, but
most physicians today agree that this regimen is unnecessary except
for patients with acute ulcers. The overall aim of dietary control, or
"physiologic rest" for the stomach which reduces mechanical, chemical and thermal trauma, is likewise questionable. However, known
stimulants of gastric secretion, such as alcohol and caffeine-containing
beverages, should be avoided. In addition, black pepper, chili powder
and mustard are direct mucosal irritants which should be eliminated.[7, 37, 44]

Small, frequent feedings provide consistent buffering effects and
avoid stimulation of gastrin due to distention.[4] All foods stimulate
production of gastric juices, but the least stimulating are carbohydrates and fats. Carbohydrates and fats, however, are the least neutral-
izing. The diet for patients with ulcers should be adequate to meet the
recommended dietary allowances yet provide an added margin of
safety to compensate for stress. Obesity should be corrected to reduce
further stress, and diets high in saturated fat should be avoided to reduce the risk of cardiovascular disease.

A strict diet for a long period of time may not only deprive the patient of needed nutrients but also may create more anxiety and stress
by eliminating most tasty foods that the patient enjoys. It is difficult for
a patient to observe a strict ulcer regimen for more than a few
weeks, and requiring observance to rigid dietary restrictions that have
not been supported by sound rationale and research adds to his diffi-
culties. On the other hand, there is always the patient with his own
beliefs about his diet.[10, 11]

CASE PRESENTATION. — V. C. is a 66-year-old man who was admitted to the
hospital with the chief complaint, "My stools are black." The patient had
wakened at 2 A.M. two days prior to admission and noted profuse perspiration.
The next morning, he passed two black, tarry stools. Stools remained black up
to the time of admission.

The patient had been seen 10 days prior to admission for evaluation for
Paget's disease. Because of back pain he was instructed to take Bufferin, 2 tab-
lets with each meal and 2 at bedtime with food. After 2 days of analgesic therapy, he began to notice vague epigastric discomfort and remembered that he
had been told 10 years previously that he had a duodenal ulcer.

An upper gastrointestinal (GI) series showed a large duodenal ulcer. The
patient was treated with antacids hourly and was instructed to avoid alcohol,
aspirin, coffee and cigarettes.

Dumping Syndrome

The "dumping" or postgastrectomy syndrome is a complication
following partial or total surgical removal of the stomach and some-

times follows drainage operations. Onset of symptoms is 10–15 minutes after ingestion of a meal and is characterized by distention followed by weakness, sweating, tachycardia, pallor, tachypnea and occasionally syncope. Normally, the intact stomach empties small quantities of food into the intestine to avoid massive and sudden changes in the osmotic load. After gastric resection, the reservoir capacity of the stomach is reduced, and ingested materials enter the intestine more rapidly and in larger quantities. Due to the increased intraluminal osmotic pressure, plasma water shifts to the intestinal lumen to equalize osmotic pressure. As a result, plasma volume drops markedly. Blood sugar levels change but do not appear to coincide with symptoms of dumping.[22]

Symptoms of the dumping syndrome are more frequently induced by carbohydrates, especially simple sugars, than by proteins and fat, and they are related to the amount of food ingested. Therefore, dietary management is of considerable importance. The basis for eliminating simple sugars and restricting carbohydrates is that the rapid hydrolysis of carbohydrates into small molecules causes the acute increase in osmotic pressure. The diet should be high in protein and fat and limited in carbohydrates, should supply 2,000–3,500 kcal/day and should include at least six feedings; fluids should be taken between meals but should be restricted with meals.

CASE PRESENTATION.—L. M. is a 45-year-old man who presented with a history of back pain. The patient said that he had been having pain in his back over the past two years. Back pain was made worse by twisting and by long periods of sitting or standing. The patient felt that he had probably lost about 1 1/2 inches in height over the past year. He had had a partial gastric resection with a Billroth II operation performed approximately five years prior to admission. Following this operation, he complained of symptoms associated with eating: shortly after eating, he would become diaphoretic, feel very weak and tremulous and would frequently have diarrhea. His symptoms were much worse if he drank milkshakes or large amounts of fluid with his meals.

Physical examination revealed that the patient was a thin man with thin skin associated with some atrophy of the subcutaneous tissue. Pertinent physical findings included a mild degree of kyphosis and tenderness to percussion over the spine.

X-rays of the lumbar and thoracic spine showed diffuse demineralization and decreased height of several thoracic vertebrae. Serum calcium was 10 mg/dl; phosphorus, 2.1 mg/dl; alkaline phosphatase, 9 mMu. Urine calcium was 50 mg/day (on an 800 mg calcium diet). An oral glucose tolerance test showed 200 mg/dl sugar at 1/2 hour, 150 mg/dl at 1 hour, 40 mg/dl at 2 hours, 60 mg/dl at 3 hours, and a gradual rise in blood sugar at 4, 5 and 6 hours. A bone biopsy showed wide osteoid seams compatible with osteomalacia and large resorption cavities compatible with osteoporosis. The pathologic interpretation was osteoporosis and osteomalacia.

The patient was placed on a high protein diet and was instructed to avoid taking fluids with meals. He improved somewhat and took calcium and vitamin D supplements.

Comment: This patient demonstrates the typical findings of dumping syndrome accompanied by malabsorption due to rapid transit. This combination of findings is frequently seen in postgastrectomy patients.

Other Complications of Gastric Surgery

Nutritional problems following gastrectomies are quite common, and the more extensive the gastric resection, the greater the nutritional problem. Patients fail to regain or maintain normal body weight, or they may lack one or more essential nutrients. Nutritional problems may arise from poor caloric intake because of "early" satiety, decreased gastric reservoir or fear of postprandial symptoms. Diarrhea, malabsorption and steatorrhea frequently result in weight loss and malnutrition. The cause of steatorrhea is somewhat controversial. Possible causes include the suggestion of decreased pancreatic secretion, rapid intestinal transit, afferent loop stasis and bacterial overgrowth.[22]

Anemia is a common complication of partial gastrectomy. Generally, a mild iron deficiency responds to oral administration of iron. Decreased serum vitamin B_{12} levels may result from impaired absorption due to decreased intrinsic factor, but megaloblastic anemia seldom develops. Coincidental, folic acid deficiency may lead to megaloblastic anemia, and chronic malabsorption of calcium and vitamin D may lead to osteoporosis and osteomalacia.

For patients with an obvious deficiency of iron, vitamin B_{12} or folic acid, these should be administered parenterally if not well absorbed. Anabolic agents and vitamin supplements should be prescribed. If steatorrhea is a grave problem, MCT may be substituted as the source of fat in the diet, and adequate calcium and vitamin D should be provided. If diarrhea is the result of bacterial overgrowth in an afferent loop with stasis, antibiotics should be administered. Again, if the dumping syndrome is a problem, the diet should be low in carbohydrate.

Nutrition in Diseases of the Intestines

Small Bowel Diseases

Signs and symptoms of malabsorption may differ as widely as the conditions that cause impaired absorption. Malabsorption of a single substance, as in poor vitamin B_{12} absorption and pernicious anemia, may be found. Similarly, celiac disease may show a defect in folic acid absorption causing megaloblastic anemia without malabsorption of fat or other substances. Patients with these conditions do not have symptoms related to the intestinal tract. On the other hand, the small bowel may be so diffusely involved that a patient has severe malabsorption with incapacitating diarrhea.

Patients may exhibit malabsorption syndromes after massive resection of the small bowel or due to a wide variety of diseases which can involve the mucosa of the small bowel (e.g., tropical and nontropical sprue, inflammatory disease and acute infections). Malabsorption of nutrients depends upon the area of the upper gastrointestinal tract involved. Table 3–1 specifies the nutrients which are most likely to be lost according to the area of the bowel involved. Malabsorption can result from a decrease in the absorptive area, damage to the mucosal epithelium, defective enzymes resulting from damage to the bowel or congenital absence of enzymes. In addition, any factor which increases motility and thus decreases the time that the intestine is exposed to its contents will decrease absorption.

In resections or diffuse processes involving up to eight feet of the proximal jejunum, malabsorption may be minimal, since protein and fat can be handled by the distal bowel. No malabsorption of folic acid, calcium, sugars, fat or fat-soluble vitamins will occur if the duodenum remains intact and transit is only minimally accelerated. However, if proximal involvement exceeds eight feet, fat and protein absorption, as well as absorption of all fat-soluble vitamins and minerals dependent upon them, are impaired. With severe ileal involvement, vitamin B_{12}, fat, fat-soluble vitamins and bile salts are lost. Vitamin B_{12} may

TABLE 3-1.—MALABSORPTION OF NUTRIENTS
ACCORDING TO AREA OF SMALL BOWEL INVOLVED

AREA OF SMALL BOWEL	NUTRIENTS	FACTORS ALTERING ABSORPTION
Proximal	Iron Calcium Fat Sugars Amino acids Fat-soluble vitamins Folic acid	Billroth II Afferent loop Jejunal resection Nontropical sprue
Middle	Sugars Amino acids Magnesium	Massive intestinal resection
Distal	Bile salts Vitamin B_{12}	Ileal resection Disease involving ileum Regional enteritis Nontropical sprue Lymphoma

also be degraded by bacterial proliferation in the bowel. Lack of absorption of bile salts in the ileum perpetuates diarrhea; increased concentrations of bile salts reaching the colon inhibit salt and water transport by the colon, thus inducing watery diarrhea.

In general, the diet should contain 3,500–4,000 kcal/day derived largely from carbohydrates and protein. Fat intake should be restricted to the minimal amount necessary for palatability. An excessive amount of fat will accentuate diarrhea, because fat is broken down by lower intestinal bacteria that release free fatty acids, which act as an irritant and an osmotic force. Medium-chain triglycerides should be substituted for the remainder of calories derived from fat. The intake of oxalate also should be restricted, since absorption of dietary oxalate in small bowel disease is increased, particularly after ileal resection. Increased absorption of dietary oxalate results in hyperoxaluria and a greater incidence of calcium oxalate stones. Vitamin and mineral supplements must be given according to the needs of the patient. The replacement of the fat-soluble vitamins presents a particularly difficult problem. The required dose is extremely variable and depends upon the severity of the malabsorption. The lack of absorption can frequently be overcome by giving pharmacologic doses. The replacement of vitamin K can be assessed by measuring the prothrombin time; and vitamin D replacement can be assessed by following serum calcium, phosphorus and alkaline phosphatase levels and measuring serum levels of 25-hydroxy-vitamin D. The adequacy of vitamin A replacement must be followed by looking for symptomatology that reflects vitamin deficiency. Water-soluble vitamins can usually be absorbed if they are given in adequate doses. Vitamin B_{12} can easily be replaced parenterally, since it is stored in the liver and need not be given frequently; that is, it can be given every 2–4 weeks.

Mineral replacement, particularly replacement of magnesium, is frequently overlooked. Magnesium deficiency is common in patients with diffuse small bowel disease, particularly those who have had ileal bypass for the treatment of obesity. Many of the magnesium salts produce diarrhea, but magnesium gluconate has been found to be efficacious, since it does not elicit this side effect. Rather large doses are required for most patients and usually range from 2 to 4 gm of magnesium daily. Calcium carbonate is a useful salt for the replacement of calcium. Again, supplementation of 1–2 gm of calcium (2–4 gm calcium carbonate) per day is usually needed.

Gluten-sensitive enteropathies call for added dietary restriction. It is the gliadin fraction of gluten that is thought to be toxic to sensitive individuals, but a gluten-free diet is necessary for treatment. Dietary

TABLE 3-2.—FOODS TO BE ELIMINATED
ON GLUTEN-FREE DIET

Wheat and rye cereals
Wheat germ
Barley
Oatmeal
Buckwheat
Noodles
Macaroni
Spaghetti
Dumplings
Bread, rolls, crackers, cookies, pastry, cake, etc., made from wheat or rye
Ry-Krisp, rusks, zwieback, pretzels
Muffins, biscuits, waffles, pancake flour, prepared mixes
Breaded foods, bread crumbs, stuffing
Meat loaf made with bread or crackers, croquettes
Canned meat dishes
Cold cuts (unless 100% pure meat)
Gravies or cream sauces thickened with wheat flour
Commercial salad dressings (except *pure* mayonnaise)
Canned soups
Cream soups (unless thickened with cream, cornstarch or potato flour)
Commercial ice cream and cones, prepared puddings and mixes
Postum, malted milk, Ovaltine, instant coffees with wheat flour added, beer, ale
Commercial candies containing cereal products

The key is to read labels on all prepared and packaged foods.

---

elimination of wheat, barley, oat and rye products dramatically re-
lieves diarrhea and steatorrhea in these patients (Table 3-2). Two
major hypotheses have been proposed to explain the toxicity of gliadin: (1) the disease may represent an immunologic reaction to the
dietary protein and (2) the disorder may be an inborn error of metabolism due to an enzyme defect in the small intestinal mucosa. It has
also been postulated that gluten activates an endogenous mechanism
of toxicity, for example, a local mucosal immune system.

CASE PRESENTATION.—J. S. is a 51-year-old man who presented with the
chief complaint of bone pain. The patient stated that over the past year he had
been experiencing a considerable amount of pain in both knees when walking. He also had deep pain in the anterior tibial region of both legs, which was
intensified by walking and slight trauma. He had experienced rather severe
back pain in the thoracic region.
   On questioning, the patient admitted to passing 2-3 stools per day for many
years. Episodically—perhaps 2-3 times a week—he would produce as many
as 6-7 stools per day. These stools were foul smelling and floated on top of
the water. He noted that diarrhea was aggravated by spaghetti and frequently
by pie crust. His weight had remained stable in the past year.
   Laboratory tests at the time of admission revealed hemoglobin, 10.4 gm/dl;

hematocrit, 33.9%; serum calcium, 6.5 mg/dl; phosphorus, 2.1 mg/dl; alkaline phosphatase, 14.4 mMu (normally less than 6); heat stable fraction, 1.9 mMu; serum iron, 33 mg/dl; iron binding capacity, 345 mg/dl; carotene, 24 μg/ml; magnesium, 1.8 mEq/L; parathyroid hormone, 210 pg/ml (normally 100–200 pg/ml); stool fat, 53 gm/24 hr. A small bowel biopsy showed blunting and flattening of the villi, infiltration of lymphocytes and plasma cells in the lamina propria. These changes were thought to be compatible with nontropical sprue. A bone biopsy from the iliac crest was diagnostic of osteomalacia.

The patient was placed on a gluten-free diet, which produced dramatic results. After 8 weeks on the diet, the patient had gained 10 lb and had had a rather marked increase in muscle strength. He was placed on 4 gm calcium lactate and 50,000 u vitamin D daily. With this regimen, serum calcium rose to 9 mg/dl; phosphorus, to 4.0 mg/dl; and alkaline phosphatase fell to 8 mMu. After three weeks of therapy, he was completely free of bone pain.

Lactase deficiency is frequently found in patients with small bowel disease. The dietary approach to this problem will be discussed later in this chapter.

Protein-losing enteropathies present a unique nutritional problem. Hypoproteinemia develops when the rate of protein loss by excretion and catabolism exceeds the rate of nitrogen reabsorption and protein synthesis. Diseases manifesting protein-losing enteropathy have no single, common etiology and pathogenesis, but patients with these diseases exhibit many of the same symptoms. These symptoms include decreased circulating and total body albumin and normal or slightly increased rate of albumin synthesis. Patients with protein-losing enteropathy may present with edema and hypoproteinemia only. Some complain of gastrointestinal problems or symptoms of hypocalcemic tetany. These patients may also have iron deficiency anemia, amino acidurias, lymphocytopenia or eosinophilia. Protein loss into the bowel may result from many diseases: lymphagiectasia, lymphoma, intestinal lipodystrophy, carcinoma, constrictive pericarditis, regional enteritis, ulcerative colitis, celiac sprue, atrophic gastritis, Menetrier's disease, nephrosis, defective gamma globulin synthesis and some amino acidurias.[22]

Intestinal lymphagiectasia commonly produces mild gastrointestinal symptoms but at times may be characterized by severe diarrhea and steatorrhea, nausea, vomiting, abdominal pain, asymmetric edema, chylous effusions, hypoalbuminemia, hypogammaglobulinemia and lymphocytopenia. Children or young adults may develop intestinal lymphagiectasia, and its diagnosis is based on increased albumin loss and markedly dilated and telangiectatic lacteals. Small bowel biopsy shows marked morphologic changes in the submucosa or serosa. Although treatment of this disease has been unsatisfactory, restriction of dietary fat to reduce the intestinal lymph flow and pressure and substitution of MCT for part of the dietary fat have been helpful.[22, 28]

Allergic gastroenteropathy has been ameliorated by eliminating milk from the diet. Symptoms accompanying hypogammaglobulinemia, hypoalbuminemia and eosinophilia were rhinitis, asthma, eczema, growth retardation, periorbital edema and anemia. Precipitating antibodies to milk were found in stools from these patients. Fecal fat tests and xylose absorption tests were within normal limits. There was radiographic evidence of mucosal edema. Corticosteroid therapy and elimination of milk reversed the protein loss and supported the hypothesis that the condition was allergic or hyperimmune.[56]

Hypogammaglobulinemia has been seen in patients with various disorders but appears to cause absorptive defects. Defective gamma-globulin synthesis leads to gastrointestinal tract lesions and consequent serum protein loss through the gastrointestinal tract. Gluten-free diets and corticosteroid therapy have shown variable results.[22]

Carbohydrate Intolerance

This condition is characterized by bloating, abdominal discomfort, nausea, vomiting and watery-acid diarrhea occurring after ingestion of the offending carbohydrate mono- or disaccharide. Although monosaccharide intolerance is rare and is present at birth, it requires immediate diagnosis and is treated by removal of glucose and galactose from the diet so the infant can survive. Fructose is substituted for the intolerable glucose and galactose. More often, carbohydrate intolerance is precipitated by offending disaccharides: lactose, sucrose, maltose or isomaltose. This intolerance may be congenital or arise from loss of activity of a specific disaccharidase(s) due to diseases of the small intestine.[5, 12]

Lactose intolerance is the most frequently reported carbohydrate intolerance, more often seen in adults as a delayed manifestation of an inherited enzyme deficiency or an acquired deficiency. Shortening of the small bowel due to surgery or increased rate of transit after gastrectomy may also be a cause. Lactose tolerance tests are good indicators of mild intolerance and show a significant correlation between the maximum rise in blood sugar during the test and the severity of symptoms.[53] It has been suggested that prolonged abstinence from milk and milk products results in lowered lactase activity. A study done by Lebenthal and associates indicated that low lactase activity occurred in 25% of the study group after age 5 and that these individuals consumed relatively small amounts of milk. The investigators suggested that perhaps intolerance really appears before adulthood in the entire white population.[35]

Many commercial formulas that contain no lactose are available for the infant with lactose intolerance.[12, 52] The adult with lactose intolerance should exclude all milk and milk products from his diet with the exception of yogurt and buttermilk, which are fermented. Some patients may tolerate cheese as well.

CASE PRESENTATION.—B. R. is a 48-year-old man who is a clerk in a clothing store. His chief complaint is back pain. The patient considered himself to be in good health until the day before admission to the hospital, when he stepped off a curb and experienced severe pain in the midthoracic area. He was seen in the emergency room and was found to have a compression fracture of the T12 vertebra and generalized skeletal demineralization. The patient admitted that he had had some discomfort in his back over the past 2–3 years, but the discomfort had not been severe enough to cause him to seek medical attention. On measurement, it was noted that he had lost one inch in height. Review of body systems revealed that this patient had a great deal of abdominal cramping and bloating and had 3–4 soft bowel movements per day. The patient had noted this pattern for many years but did not consider it particularly abnormal.

Physical examination revealed a thin, white male in no acute distress. The skin appeared thin with loss of subcutaneous tissue. The only other abnormal finding was tenderness to percussion over the long bones.

Laboratory work showed hemoglobin, 13.9 gm/dl; normal white blood cell count; serum calcium, 8.2 mg/dl; serum phosphorus, 1.9 mg/dl; and alkaline phosphatase, 8 mMu. Upper GI series with small bowel pattern was normal. Lactose tolerance test showed no rise in serum glucose after loading with 100 gm of lactose. During this test, the patient experienced rather severe cramping, abdominal pain and diarrhea. Bone biopsy showed osteomalacia.

The diagnosis of this patient was osteomalacia secondary to lactase deficiency. The patient was placed on a lactose-free diet supplemented with calcium. He experienced marked relief of bone pain, and the alkaline phosphatase decreased to normal. Diarrhea subsided completely, and it was felt that the patient was malabsorbing calcium due to the osmotic diarrhea produced by lactose.

Acute Infectious Diarrheas

These diarrheas include salmonellosis, shigellosis, typhoid fever, cholera, infantile diarrhea, *Escherichia coli* diarrhea in adults, viral gastroenteritis, staphylococcal food poisoning and dysentery. Generally, the diarrhea is "explosive," with a consequent loss of fluid and electrolytes. Therapy is directed toward maintenance of fluid and electrolyte balance, good nutrition and elimination of the causative microorganism.

Salmonellosis and shigellosis are probably the more common causes of infectious gastroenteritis in this country. Mucosal changes are most pronounced in the terminal ileum from *Salmonella* invasion. Mucosal changes can alter absorption of fats and fat-soluble vitamins and other nutrients. Shigellosis mainly affects the colon with lesions ranging from congestion and erythema to ulceration and perforation.[22]

Cholera is caused by the organism *Vibrio cholerae* and is a full-blown form of infectious diarrhea particularly prevalent in malnourished populations. Profuse, watery diarrhea isotonic with plasma is the major symptom. Patients are generally afebrile and continue to have diarrhea for approximately four days. Vomiting and skeletal muscle cramping are early secondary effects of marked electrolyte imbalance. The mortality rate is quite high for untreated patients; however, adequate treatment lowers the mortality rate to almost zero. Oral administration of glucose and bicarbonate, potassium, sodium and chloride in concentrations equal to those in the stool stimulates absorption of intestinal fluid and leads to an immediate decrease in the volume of stools. If dumping occurs, fluid replacement must be given intravenously. Tetracycline usually shortens the duration of the disease.[22]

Regional Enteritis

Dawson described several nutritional disturbances associated with regional enteritis.[16] Intake of food is poor due to anorexia associated with ill-health and the fear of more abdominal pain. Iron deficiency anemia may result from blood loss and poor absorption, while anemia due to folate deficiency results from poor intake and impaired absorption. Uptake of vitamin B_{12} may be impaired due to the disease, resection of the ileum or bacterial proliferation. Bile salt reabsorption may be impaired as a result of degradation of bile salts by colonic bacteria or resection of the ileum (site of reabsorption). Hypoproteinemia may result from excessive loss of protein from the inflamed bowel. Electrolyte losses, dehydration and fat-soluble vitamin losses accompany steatorrhea.

A diet low in fat has been suggested by several investigators.[16, 38, 40] The low fat diet reduces the load on the diminished absorptive capacity of the bowel and prevents loss of fat in the stool leading to improved absorption of other nutrients. Fat restriction also limits the formation of free fatty acids, which increase diarrhea by mechanisms already described. For patients with regional ileitis, a low residue diet to reduce bolus colic in strictured areas of the small bowel has been suggested.[38] However, Manier found no evidence of any beneficial effect from the low residue diet.[40] A high protein high calorie diet is necessary if fever, malabsorption or protein loss occurs.

Ulcerative Colitis

Ulcerative colitis is of unknown etiology and is characterized by exacerbation and remission. Abdominal pain, diarrhea, rectal bleeding, weight loss and debilitation are some of its symptoms. The mucosa is more diffusely and uniformly granular and friable than in regional enteritis. Again, malnutrition is common due to losses, decreased intake, dehydration and steatorrhea.

Manier pointed out the lack of evidence of beneficial effect from a low residue diet for ulcerative colitis. Others feel that there is no evidence against the low residue diet.[40] Again, the diet should be high in protein and calories; patients with milk intolerance due to an immunologic mechanism or to lactase depletion secondary to the disease process should avoid milk. Liquid elemental diets have had positive results, including weight gain, healed areas of ulceration and positive nitrogen balance[8, 9] (see Table 6–1). Many of the same medications used in the treatment of regional enteritis are employed in the control of ulcerative colitis.

CASE PRESENTATION.—A. B. is a 27-year-old woman who presented with the chief complaint of diarrhea. The patient stated that 4 weeks prior to admission, she noticed bloody mucus on the outside of her stools. Over the next four weeks, she developed cramping lower abdominal pain and diarrhea with 8–10 stools daily. Diarrhea occurred at night as well as during the day. She lost 6 lb.

Physical examination revealed a pale, weak-appearing woman. Her height was 157.5 cm; weight, 49 kg. There was tenderness to palpatation over the left colon and no abnormalities of the skin or joints. Proctosigmoidoscopy revealed a red and edematous mucosa with a pitted, granular appearance. The mucosa bled easily and was covered with a mucopurulent exudate.

The patient was placed on a liquid elemental diet, Vivonex, to reduce stimulation of colonic activity. Sedatives and corticosteroids were prescribed. As symptoms subsided and the appearance of the colonic mucosa improved, the diet was gradually liberalized. Over a period of months, the patient was placed on a relatively normal diet that excluded milk and raw vegetables.

Other Colonic Diseases

Diverticulosis, diverticulitis and constipation have been associated with the refined carbohydrate diet of Western civilization. Several investigators have suggested that diverticulae form from isolated segments of high intracolonic pressures due to small fecal mass accompanying a diet low in bulk.[15, 20, 40, 45, 46, 47]

Diverticulosis generally presents few if any nutritional complications. However, accumulation of fecal matter in the pockets along the colon often causes inflammation, formation of abscesses or fistulae, perforation or obstruction. This condition is diverticulitis, which is treated more cautiously.

CASE PRESENTATION.—M. F. is a 60-year-old man who presented with severe lower abdominal pain, fever and vomiting. He had a long history of cramping abdominal pain and had been diagnosed as having diverticulitis. He had been on a low residue diet for several years and had noted recurrence of symptoms after eating nuts or popcorn. His present problem had begun with an increase of abdominal cramping and progression of symptoms about 3 days prior to admission to the hospital.

Physical examination revealed a well-developed, moderately obese man in acute distress, with temperature, 38 C; pulse, 100 beats/min, blood pressure, 120/70 mmHg, clear chest. The abdomen was distended and tenderness diffuse throughout, with more marked findings—rebound tenderness—in the left lower quadrant. X-ray examination revealed a mass in the lower left quadrant surrounding the colon and representing abscess formation around a ruptured diverticulum. A transverse colostomy was performed for decompression and diversion of fecal material, and antibiotics and intravenous fluid therapy were instituted. Two months later, the transverse colon was reanastomosed, and a short segment of the sigmoid colon was removed.

The patient followed a low residue diet for about six months and continued to experience episodes of cramping abdominal pain. He was then placed on a high fiber diet and noted improvement in symptoms.

Manier suggested a high residue diet, plus large amounts of hydroscopic colloids, to prevent apposition of the colonic wall and development of high pressure segments.[40] Goldstein supported this view, suggesting that the traditional low residue diets increase the problem for patients with diverticulosis.[20, 21] An unrefined diet of adequate fiber may prevent diverticulosis, since the colon must cope with a large volume of feces with less time for water absorption. Painter found that bran relieved or abolished abdominal aching, pain and distention.[45, 46]

Diverticulitis must sometimes be treated by surgery, especially if perforation occurs. If diverticulitis is treated medically, a low fiber diet has usually been prescribed. However, a low fiber diet may lead to further formation of diverticulae. Most patients have learned by "trial and error" which foods they must avoid to prevent irritation and bleeding. Generally, the elimination of nuts, corn and seeds, which manage to lodge in the diverticulae, is adequate dietary management.

Constipation is becoming an exceedingly common disorder; it is more of a symptom than a disease and usually results from production of abnormally hard and dry stools, suppression of defecation and inadequate quantity of stool. The most common inorganic cause of colonic constipation is probably inadequate dietary residue and water intake. The major cause of both rectal and colonic constipation is drugs, especially opiates, anticholinergic agents, ganglionic blockers, nonabsorbable antacids, antidepressants, sedatives and anti-Parkinsonian agents.[6] Constipation should be treated by dealing with its cause. If the problem is related to poor habits or an inadequate diet, the patient should be carefully advised.

Particularly in the elderly, the amount of the soft bulk residue in the diet should be increased initially through cooked vegetables and canned or stewed fruits. As bowel movements improve, fresh fruits and vegetables and bran should be added. Prunes stimulate peristalsis and contain fiber. In addition, figs, applesauce, bananas, whole grain cereals and bread containing bran provide adequate residue. Bran shortens transit time.[6] Adequate fluid intake, at least 1,500 ml daily, is also important. Cheese, chocolate, tea and sometimes coffee may be constipating and should therefore be avoided. Laxatives should be prescribed only if absolutely necessary and if the patient can be carefully observed. Laxatives classed in order of their increasing action are lubricants, bulk-forming agents, saline cathartics and stimulants. Although the bulk-forming agents are probably the safest to use, hazards, such as allergic reactions and inspissation in the esophagus, may result if the amount of water taken with these agents is not adequate.[6]

Nutrition in Diseases of the Liver

Diet therapy is one of the most important aspects in the management of patients with diseases of the liver. Although there is little scientific evidence for this form of therapy, diet therapy has been adhered to over the years and has proved essential to treat such complications as ascites and hepatic coma. A great deal of controversy has arisen over the role of diet and pathogenesis of hepatic diseases. Although it is agreed that malnutrition can produce liver changes in kwashiorkor and other forms of fatty liver, it is denied by many that cirrhosis in man is caused by nutritional injury alone. In general, the objective of diet therapy is to protect the liver from stress and to enable the damaged liver to function as easily and efficiently as possible.

Viral Hepatitis

Infectious hepatitis is the most common hepatic disease seen in Western civilization, but other viruses may also cause liver disease. Bacteria, such as brucellosis, spirochetes, such as syphilis, fungi, such as histoplasmosis, protozoa, such as amebiasis, and helminths, such as schistosomiasis, may also cause liver disease.[22]

Often patients with viral hepatitis experience anorexia, nausea, vomiting and diarrhea resulting in limitations in food and fluid intake. Gabuzda recommended a progression in diet therapy: First, if oral intake is less than 15–20 kcal/kg/day, 10% glucose in water should be given intravenously as a source of calories, and B-complex vitamins should be added. When the appetite has begun to return, small, "bland" feedings may be tolerated. With amelioration of symptoms, an intake of 25–30 kcal/kg/day with 0.5–1.0 gm protein/kg/day should be achieved in 4–6 small, well-balanced meals (dietary fat restricted during period of cholestasis). The diet should be gradually increased to 1.0 gm protein/kg/day with 35–40 kcal/kg/day and moderate fat.[19] The small, frequent feedings satisfy the patient's hunger and tend to reduce the anorexia and severe nausea that appear with fewer and larger meals. Milkshakes and eggnogs for interval feedings supply a good source of protein and calories, and they are well tolerated by these patients. Supplements are also commercially available.

If oral intake does not ensure an adequate intake of nutrients, tube feedings must be considered. Many commercially available tube-feeding formulas would be appropriate (see Chapter 6). If, because of complications, such as ascites or impending hepatic coma, a severe restriction in sodium and/or protein is needed, the tube-feeding preparation may have to be developed by a dietitian, who can calculate a diet that provides adequate calories and the necessary restrictions.

A few comments regarding the three major nutrients—protein, fat and carbohydrate—might be appropriate at this point. Protein should come from both animal and vegetable sources to assure adequate supplies of total protein, choline, inositol, methionine, other amino acids and vitamins. Meats, fish, eggs, dairy products and cereals are such sources. Amino acid supplements are not necessary if digestion and absorption are not impaired; vitamin supplements are unnecessary unless food intake is poor. Fat restriction is unnecessary for patients with infectious hepatitis, unless it causes digestive disturbances. High fat diets may provoke steatorrhea and/or anorexia and nausea.[36] However, a diet with 30–40% of the calories derived from fat adds palatability, carries the fat-soluble vitamins and is well tolerated especially during convalescence. Since foods high in protein are also generally high in fat, the diet is much easier to plan and enjoy. Carbohydrate is readily obtained in a well-balanced diet. In fact, it is the least of the dietitian's worries when planning a diet for these patients. It is not necessary to incorporate hard candy and desserts in these diets;

these items usually inhibit the appetite for nutritiously balanced foods.

When intrahepatic biliary obstruction occurs in patients with infectious hepatitis, exclusion of bile from the gut may interfere with absorption of fats and vitamin K. Plasma prothrombin levels are often reduced as a result of poor absorption of vitamin K and the inability of the liver to synthesize prothrombin. Usually, parenteral vitamin K or oral, water-soluble vitamin K will effectively raise prothrombin levels. The degree of response depends upon hepatic function, which in itself is a good test for impairment of liver function.

Complications of infectious hepatitis, such as hepatic coma and cirrhosis, require modifications of dietary management.

Hepatic Coma

Hepatic coma is a very complex pathophysiologic state that can be aggravated by many different factors. In the presence of severe impairment of hepatic function, the patient becomes unable to detoxify the metabolic products of protein degraded by the bacteria in the intestinal tract; therefore, any increased protein load, whether dietary in origin or due to blood in the gastrointestinal tract, is very poorly tolerated. The development of metabolic alkalosis also tends to increase the symptoms of encephalopathy.

Toxic substances that are known to accumulate in hepatic failure and can be shown to produce reversible coma in experimental animals are ammonia, fatty acids and mercaptans. The effects of these substances appear to be interdependent; markedly reduced blood levels of these substances induce coma in normal animals when any two of them are injected simultaneously. There is a very good correlation between the urinary concentration of mercaptans, particularly methanethiol, and the development of hepatic coma. It has also been shown by Zieve that fetor hepaticus is probably due to pulmonary excretion of a mixture of a methanethiol, dimethylsulfide and dimethyldisulfide.[58]

The patient with severe hepatic disease must be observed carefully for signs of impending hepatic coma, and diet must be altered for patients who show clinical signs of hepatic failure. These patients have a very poor tolerance for protein, particularly proteins with large quantities of sulfur-containing amino acids such as animal protein. Greenberger recently has presented evidence that patients who are in danger of impending coma do much better if the major source of their dietary protein comes from vegetables, which reduces the intake of sulfur-containing amino acids.[22a] Protein intake should be restricted to less than 0.5 mg/kg/day for patients with hepatic encephalopathy, and more severe restriction is required for those who are in a coma. Administration of the amino acids that stimulate the urea cycle—arginine, aspartate and glutamate—may be helpful in lowering serum ammonia levels. Acidification with arginine hydrochloride has also been shown to decrease serum ammonia levels. Antibiotic therapy to sterilize the gut helps decrease protein degradation by gut bacteria.[59]

Fatty Liver

In association with kwashiorkor, pellagra, ulcerative colitis, tuberculosis and alcoholism, fatty liver is well known. Although many believe that fatty liver is the forerunner of cirrhosis, the progression of fatty liver to cirrhosis is still questionable. Toxic factors may cause hepatic cellular necrosis or autoimmune responses which cause further damage. If cirrhosis developed as a result of nutritional deficiency alone, an adequate, well-balanced diet would prevent fatty liver from becoming cirrhotic. However, it does not appear to be so simple.

It has been assumed for many years that the accumulation of fat in the liver of alcoholics was based on nutritional deficiency, especially the deficiency of protein, choline and methionine. However, the metabolic effects of alcohol must be considered. Large amounts of alcohol have been shown to cause translocation of fat from adipose tissue to the liver in the same way as stressful situations. Amounts of alcohol equal to the usual alcoholic's intake tend to increase the synthesis of fat in the liver. When alcohol was substituted for sucrose in an adequate diet, fatty change in the liver was induced.[55]

Toxic Hepatitis and Cirrhosis

The management of acute toxic hepatitis should be similar to that of infectious hepatitis. Dietary management has been shown to enhance resistance to and repair of hepatic damage by toxic agents, such as carbon tetrachloride. Some oral contraceptives, psychochemotherapeutic agents and other drugs may lead to iatrogenic jaundice. Other toxic liver diseases such as Senecio cirrhosis seen in South African and North American cattle, have been related to nutritional factors. Senecio is a plant that grows in the wheat fields of Cape Province. Its crushed seeds may be turned into flour and thereby contaminate bread and other foods made from the flour. If animals and men have an adequate protein intake, they seem to be protected from this disease.[22]

Diet therapy for patients with cirrhosis is not always successful.

Some alcoholics with Laennec's cirrhosis have been restored to and kept in good health by diet therapy in combination with avoidance of alcohol. However, many more patients with cirrhosis die from hepatic failure or bleeding esophageal varices.[22]

For patients with uncomplicated hepatic cirrhosis, diet may be given ad libitum, and protein tolerance can vary in different patients. Gabuzda recommends 25–30 kcal/kg/day and 0.7 gm protein/kg/day initially. Then, unless neuropsychiatric symptoms develop, 10–15 gm protein and 200–300 kcal/kg/day can be added at 5–7-day intervals. The goal is to achieve a total intake of 1 gm protein/kg/day and 25–40 kcal/kg/day.[19, 55]

Edema and ascites are common complications of cirrhosis and are usually associated with malnutrition, endocrinologic problems and secondary metabolic changes. Loss of muscle mass and a raw, beefy tongue are due to protein waste and vitamin B-complex deficiency. Scurvy, pellagra, cheilosis and other signs of vitamin B-complex deficiency may be seen. Spider nevi, liver palms, loss of libido, testicular and prostatic atrophy, loss of hair on the chest, gynecomastia and amenorrhea or menorrhagia are the usual endocrinologic changes and are related to the abnormal production and degradation of hormones. Hormonal aberrations may be due to malnutrition and/or the inability of the damaged liver to conjugate and deactivate normally circulating hormones. The metabolic defects are hypoalbuminemia, electrolyte imbalance, decreased levels of prothrombin and cholinesterase in the serum.[22]

Water retention has been associated with increased portal pressure, hypoalbuminemia, increased antidiuretic hormone, secondary aldosteronism and tissue permeability. Salt and water in the diet expand extracellular fluid volume isotonically in patients with liver disease; so weight gain is directly proportional to sodium intake. Gabuzda recommends initial treatment with a diet of 250 mg sodium, 50 gm protein, about 2,000 kcal and 1,500 ml fluid per day. Long-term management consists of a well-balanced diet restricted in sodium. When ascites and edema are no longer evident, sodium restriction should be continued for several weeks to a month. Then a gradual, daily increment of 500 to 1,000 mg sodium should be tolerated. Daily sodium intake for these patients should never exceed 2,500 mg.[19]

Host and associates have described the use of hyperalimentation of patients with cirrhosis. This form of diet therapy is generally a last resort. A solution of synthetic amino acids (4.1 gm essential and nonessential amino acids), 20 gm glucose, up to 0.1 mEq K^+, 0.8 mEq Na^+ and 55–70 μg ammonia/100 ml was given to cirrhotic patients and carefully observed. This therapy was advantageous because of the strict sodium and ammonia control, but it caused an unexplained rise in some liver enzymes. However, these enzymes returned toward normal as treatment continued and the patients improved. Portal pressures remained unchanged by infusion of large volumes of the solution. Ammonia levels rose modestly but without signs of hepatic encephalopathy.[29]

Cholecystitis and Gallstones

Cholecystitis is not an infectious disease but is the result of chemical inflammation of the wall of the gallbladder. However, secondary bacterial infection and ischemia may develop. The predisposition to gallstones as a result of diet and obesity remains controversial due to various independent studies in different parts of the world. More research is needed to link certain dietary patterns, such as those high in saturated or unsaturated fat or those high in refined carbohydrate, with cholelithiasis.[14, 17]

A prerequisite to the formation of gallstones composed primarily of cholesterol is bile saturated with cholesterol. Increased hepatic synthesis and biliary secretion of cholesterol is combined with decreased hepatic synthesis of bile acids and size of the bile-acid pool in patients with cholelithiasis. Crystallization may be induced by mucoproteins, refluxed intestinal contents, bile pigments, foreign bodies or bacteria. The rate of stone formation may also be influenced by efficiency of gallbladder emptying and selective absorption of lipids by the gallbladder.[14]

Dietary management of patients with gallstones and cholecystitis is primarily empirical. A time-honored dietary regimen is the prescribed low fat diet. Greasy or fried foods, eggs, mayonnaise, salad dressings, cheese and pork products and high fat-containing pastries rich in cream should be avoided. In addition, about half the patients with gallstones recognize they cannot tolerate onions, sauerkraut, cabbage, radishes, turnips, cucumbers and spicy foods.[22] Dietary management has not currently been discussed in the literature.

Chronic Obstructive Jaundice

This form of liver disease is commonly seen as a result of undetected calculi, cholangiolitis, biliary cirrhosis, postoperative traumatic stricture or congenital lesions of the bile ducts, carcinoma of the pancreas or hepatic ducts and cysts in the head of the pancreas. Steatorrhea is the main pathophysiologic disturbance resulting in malnutrition due to loss of calories, fat-soluble vitamins and minerals. Steatorrhea may lead to development of fatty liver and impaired production of plasma proteins. Medium-chain triglycerides are better absorbed, since they do not require micelle formation with bile. Failure to absorb vitamin K leads to prothrombin deficiency noted by spontaneous bruising and hemorrhagic tendencies. Loss of calcium and vitamin D produces osteomalacia leading to fractures, collapse of vertebrae and herniation of the intervertebral disc. Osteoporosis may develop from protein and calcium deficiency. Night blindness and hyperkeratosis is produced by vitamin A deficiency. Failure to absorb unsaturated fatty acids may cause eczematous skin lesions. Loss of potassium may cause potassium nephropathy, atony of the bowel and muscle weakness.[22, 27, 28]

In addition to providing MCT, the diet should be restricted to 40 gm fat daily, most from food sources rich in protein. Sufficient calories should be provided in the regimen. Vitamin K may have to be given by intramuscular injection until the deficiency is corrected. Vitamin D may have to be taken in massive doses if bone lesions are present. Calcium supplements should be taken in addition to skim milk, buttermilk and other high calcium low-fat foods. If anemia is present, the vitamin B complex and vitamin B_{12} are first prescribed. If no response is noted, ferrous sulfate should be added. Intravenous iron therapy or transfusions may be necessary in some instances.[22] If cirrhosis develops, the dietary management described previously is necessary.

REFERENCES

1. Abraham, S.: Effect of diet on hepatic fatty acid synthesis, J. Am. Diet. Assoc. 23:1120, 1970.
2. Adibi, S. A., Fogel, M. R., and Radheshyam, M. A.: Comparison of free amino acid and dipeptide absorption in the jejunum of sprue patients, Gastroenterology 67:586, 1974.
3. Allan, R., et al.: Changes in the bidirectional sodium flux across the intestinal mucosa in Crohn's disease, Gut 16:201, 1975.
4. Babouris, N., Fletcher, J., and Lennard-Jones, J. E.: Effect of varying the size and frequency of meals, Gut 6:118,1965.
5. Bayless, T. M.: Disaccharidase deficiency, J. Am. Diet. Assoc. 60:478, 1972.
6. Benson, J. A.: Simple chronic constipation, Postgrad. Med. 57:55, 1975.
7. Buchman, E., Kaung, D. T., and Knapp, R. N.: Dietary treatment in duodenal ulcer, Am. J. Clin. Nutr. 22:1536, 1969.
8. Bury, K. D., Stephens, R. V., and Randall, H. T.: Use of a chemically defined, liquid, elemental diet for nutritional management of fistulas of the alimentary tract, Am. J. Surg. 1210:174, 1971.
9. Bury, K. D., Turnier, E., and Randall, H. T.: Nutritional management of granulomatous colitis with perineal ulceration, Can. J. Surg. 15:108, 1972.

10. Caron, H. S., and Roth, H. P.: Popular beliefs about the peptic ulcer diet, J. Am. Diet. Assoc. 60:306, 1972.
11. Cheraskin, E., and Ringsdorf, W. M.: Reported gastrointestinal symptoms and signs before and after dietary counsel, J. Med. Assoc. State Ala. 41:21, 1971.
12. Cocco, A. E., Gokim, G. C., and Carbary, B. J.: Disaccharide intolerance: A review for practicing physicians, Md. State Med. J. 19:51, 1970.
13. Cohen, M. I., and Gartner, L. M.: The use of medium-chain triglycerides in the management of biliary atresia, J. Pediatr. 79:379, 1971.
14. Coyne, M. J., and Schoenfield, L. J.: Gallstone disease, Postgrad. Med. 57:153, 1975.
15. Cummings, J. H.: Dietary fibre, Gut 14:69, 1973.
16. Dawson, A. M.: Nutritional disturbances in Crohn's disease, Proc. R. Soc. Med. 64:166, 1971.
17. Eastwood, M. A., Mowbray, S. L., Thompson, R. P. H., and Williams, R.: Dietary fibre and the pruritus of cholestatic jaundice, Br. J. Nutr. 24: 1029, 1970.
18. Farmer, R. G.: The protean manifestations of Crohn's disease, Postgrad. Med. 57:129, 1975.
19. Gabuzda, G. J.: Nutrition and liver disease, Med. Clin. North Am. 54: 1455, 1970.
20. Goldstein, F.: Diet and colonic disease, J. Am. Diet. Assoc. 60:499, 1972.
21. Goldstein, F.: Physiologic management of functional GI disorders, Med. Counterpoint 3:16, 1971.
22. Goodhart, R. S., and Shils, M. E.: *Modern Nutrition in Health and Disease, Dietotherapy* (5th ed.; Philadelphia: Lea & Febiger, 1973).
22a. Greenberger, N. J.: Personal communication.
23. Grundy, D. J.: Small bowel fistula treated with low residue diet, Br. Med. J. 2:531, 1971.
24. Haig, T. H.: Pancreatic digestive enzymes: Influence of a diet that augments pancreatitis, J. Surg. Res. 10:601, 1970.
25. Hill, G. L., et al.: Effect of a chemically defined liquid elemental diet on composition and volume of ileal fistula drainage, Gastroenterology 68: 676, 1975.
26. Hofmann, A. F., and Poley, J. R.: Role of bile acid malabsorption in pathogenesis of diarrhea and steatorrhea in patients with ileal resection, I. Response to cholestyramine or replacement of dietary long-chain triglyceride by medium-chain triglyceride, Gastroenterology 62:918, 1972.
27. Holt, P. R.: Fats and bile salts, II. Pathologic considerations, J. Am. Diet. Assoc. 60:495–498, 1972.
28. Holt, P. R.: Medium-Chain Triglycerides, in Dowling, H. F. (ed.): *Disease-a-Month* (Chicago: Year Book Medical Publishers, Inc., June 1971).
29. Host, W. R., Serlin, O., and Rush, B. F.: Hyperalimentation in cirrhotic patients, Am. J. Surg. 123:57, 1972.
30. Isenberg, J. I.: Peptic ulcer disease, Postgrad. Med. 57:163, 1975.
31. Isenberg, J. I.: Therapy of peptic ulcer, J.A.M.A. 233:540, 1975.
32. Ivey, K. J.: Current concepts on physiologic control of gastric acid secretion. Clinical applications, Am. J. Med. 58:389, 1975.

33. Kettering, R. F.: Current concepts in the medical treatment of duodenal ulcer, Surg. Clin. North Am. 51:835, 1971.
34. Knowlessar, O. D.: Dietary gluten sensitivity updated, J. Am. Diet. Assoc. 60:475, 1972.
35. Lebenthal, E., Antonowicz, I., and Shwachman, H.: Correlation of lactase activity, lactose tolerance and milk consumption in different age groups, Am. J. Clin. Nutr. 28:595, 1975.
36. Leevy, C. M.: Liver disease of the alcoholic, Viewpoints on Digestive Diseases, 3:1, 1971.
37. Lennard-Jones, J. E., and Babouris, N.: Effect of different foods on the acidity of the gastric contents in patients with duodenal ulcer. I. A comparison between two 'therapeutic' diets and freely chosen meals, Gut 6:113, 1965.
38. Lennard-Jones, J. E., and Morson, B. C.: Changing Concepts in Crohn's Disease, in Dowling., H. F. (ed.): *Disease-a-Month* (Chicago: Year Book Medical Publishers, Inc., August 1969).
39. Lifshitz, F., Coello-Ramirez, P., Gutierrez-Topete, G., and Cornado-Cornet, M. C.: Carbohydrate intolerance in infants with diarrhea, J. Pediatr. 79:760, 1971.
40. Manier, J. W.: Diet in gastrointestinal diseases, Med. Clin. North Am. 54:1357, 1970.
41. Moberg, S., and Carlberger, G.: The effect on gastric emptying of test meals with various fat and osmolar concentrations, Scand. J. Gastroenterol. 9:29, 1974.
42. Moberg, S., Carlberger, G., and Barany, F.: Digestion and absorption in the duodenum in relation to gastric emptying in a patient with duodenal ulcer; methodological and physiological considerations, Scand. J. Gastroenterol. 9:9, 1974.
43. Mulcare, D. B., Dennin, H. F., and Drenick, E. J.: Effect of diet on malabsorption after small bowel bypass, J. Am. Diet. Assoc. 57:331, 1970.
44. Odell, A. C.: Ulcer dietotherapy—past and present, J. Am. Diet. Assoc. 58:447, 1971.
45. Painter, N. S.: Irritable or irritated bowel, Br. Med. J. 2:46, 1972.
46. Painter, N. S., Almeida, A. Z., and Colebourne, K. W.: Unprocessed bran in treatment of diverticular disease of the colon, Br. Med. J. 2:137, 1972.
47. Painter, N. S., and Burkitt, D. P.: Diverticular disease of the colon: A deficiency disease of western civilization, Br. Med. J. 2:450, 1971.
48. Payler, D. K., et al.: The effect of wheat bran on intestinal transit, Gut 16:209, 1975.
49. Raha, P. K., Sengupta, K. P., and Aikat, B. K.: Chronic cholecystitis and cholelithiasis: An experimental study, Indian J. Med. Res. 59:873, 1971.
50. Rudman, D., Galambos, J. T., Wenger, J., and Achord, J. L.: Adverse effects of dietary gluten in four patients with regional enteritis, Am. J. Clin. Nutr. 24:1068, 1971.
51. Sarles, H., Crotte, C., Gerolami, A., Mule, A., Domingo, N., and Hauton, J.: The influence of calorie intake and of dietary protein on the bile lipids, Scand. J. Gastroenterol. 6:189, 1971.
52. Skala, I., and Lamacova, V.: Diets in lactose intolerance, Nutr. Metab. 13:200, 1971.

53. Stephenson, L. S., and Latham, M. C.: Lactose tolerance tests as a predictor of milk tolerance, Am. J. Clin. Nutr. 28:86, 1975.
54. Strober, W., et al.: The pathogenesis of gluten-sensitive enteropathy, Ann. Intern. Med. 83:242, 1975.
55. Symposium: Nutrition and liver injury, I and II, Am. J. Clin. Nutr. 23: 447, 581, 1970.
56. Waldmann, T. A., et al.: Allergic gastroenteropathy. A cause of excessive gastrointestinal protein loss, N. Engl. J. Med. 276:762, 1967.
57. West, R. J., and Lloyd, J. K.: The effect of cholestyramine on intestinal absorption, Gut 16:93, 1975.
58. Zieve, L., Doizak, W. M., and Zieve, F. J.: Synergism between mercaptans and ammonia or fatty acids in the production of coma: A possible role for mercaptans in the pathogenesis of hepatic coma, J. Lab. Clin. Med. 83:16, 1974.
59. Zieve, L., and Nicoloff, D. M.: Pathogenesis of hepatic coma, Annu. Rev. Med. 26:143, 1975.

Chapter 4 / Nutrition in Endocrinology and Metabolism

Diabetes

NUTRITIONAL FACTORS are among the important determinants of the prevalence of diabetes. Twelve age-matched populations of 11 countries in Central America and the United States were tested by standardized methods to determine the association between the prevalence of hyperglycemia and certain epidemiologic variables, including several nutritional factors.[41] In general, the association between the prevalence of diabetes and the dietary intake of fat and sugar was positive. Conversely, the association between the prevalence of diabetes and total carbohydrate consumption was negative. There were some inconsistencies in these associations, but the trend was apparent. The most impressive and consistent association was between the prevalence of diabetes and obesity. In terms of prevention, then, the maintenance of ideal body weight is by far the most important factor known at this time.

Recommendations for the composition of a diabetic diet have varied from Ebers Parchment's recommendations of wheat grains, honey, berries and sweet beer as medicines "to drive away the passing of too much urine" to the recommendations of John Rollo, the Surgeon General of Royal Artillery in the English Army in 1797, which ushered in an era of complete avoidance of dietary carbohydrate to eliminate sugar from the urine. Bouchardat, the noted French clinician, set forth as a second major principle in the dietary education of diabetics to eat as little as possible and periodically fast for the purpose of controlling glucosuria. In the late 1800s, a German, Naunyn, introduced the term "acidosis" and discovered that sugar could also be made from protein. He therefore recommended that both sugar and protein be eliminated from the diet. Following in his footsteps, Fredrick M. Allen, M.D., of the Rockefeller Institute introduced the famous "Allen's starvation treatment." Using this treatment, several young men lived for a number of years on 10 gm of carbohydrate and 1,000 kcal/day. Although emaciated and so weak that they could not get out of bed, these men were able to survive until the advent of insulin. A low carbohydrate, high fat, calorically restricted diet was then the cornerstone of diabetic therapy from the time of Rollo until the discovery of insulin. A Dutchman, Von Noorden, kept alive the concept of a high carbohydrate diet by introducing the "oat cure" in 1902. He was joined by several other clinicians, who recommended a high carbohydrate diet consisting of rice, potatoes, milk and oatmeal.

The effect of high carbohydrate diets for patients with mild diabetes was studied more recently by Brunzell.[3] Glucose and immunoreactive insulin levels were measured in normal persons and subjects with mild diabetes maintained on a 45 or 85% carbohydrate formula diet. Fasting glucose levels fell in all subjects, and oral glucose tolerance tests significantly improved after ten days of high carbohydrate feeding. Fasting insulin levels were lower on the high carbohydrate diet, but insulin response to oral glucose did not change significantly. It was suggested that high carbohydrate diets increased the sensitivity of peripheral tissues to insulin.

One of the major disadvantages of strict carbohydrate restriction is that much of the caloric deficit must be made up by fat. In view of the high incidence of atherosclerosis in diabetic patients, restricting cholesterol and saturated fat would seem more reasonable. On the other hand, it is important to remember that type IV hyperlipoproteinemia is common in diabetics, and carbohydrates should be restricted for these patients.

The question has been raised as to whether or not sorbitol and mannitol could be substituted for sucrose and glucose for diabetics. Sharkey studied the metabolism of sorbitol and mannitol in diabetic subjects.[35] Sorbitol is an alcohol commercially made from glucose by hydrogenation, and it occurs naturally in many fruits and vegetables. Sorbitol is wholly absorbed into the blood stream and apparently is metabolized without insulin. It has the same caloric value as glucose. Mannitol is extracted commercially from sea-tangle (Laminaria) and is also the main constituent of mannose. It can be obtained commercially by hydrogenation of mannose and is found in some fruits and vegetables. Mannitol supplies half the caloric value of glucose. Sixty-five percent of the ingested mannitol is absorbed slowly, and one third of the absorbed mannitol is excreted intact in the urine; the remainder is oxidized by the liver.

Current opinion concerning ideal composition of a diabetic diet is summarized in the statement of the Committee on Food and Nutrition: "There no longer appears to be a need to restrict disproportionately the intake of carbohydrates in the diet of most diabetic patients. Increase of dietary carbohydrate even to extremes without increase of total calories does not appear to increase insulin requirement in the insulin-treated diabetic patient. The average proportion of calories consumed as carbohydrates in U. S. population as a whole approximates 45%. This proportion or even higher appears to be acceptable for the usual diabetic patient as well."[5] Recently, some researchers have recommended that the diabetic diet should be high in fiber. Jenkins reported a marked reduction in insulin requirements when large quantities of raw vegetables were added to the diet.[22]

In retrospect, the common thread running through all diabetic diets prescribed since ancient times has been caloric restriction. The debate continues as to whether high or low carbohydrate diets improve glucose tolerance. One must keep in mind that the therapeutic objectives of dietary control of diabetes are to *obtain ideal body weight, control glycosuria and prevent ketosis.*

CASE PRESENTATION. – K. T. is a 20-year-old woman who has had diabetes mellitus since the age of 11. She was hospitalized because of poor control of the disease. The patient previously had been placed on a 1,500 kcal diet, which included a feeding at bedtime; insulin dosage had been 40 units isophane insulin (NPH) with 15 units of regular insulin in the morning and 15 units NPH with 10 units regular insulin in the evening before supper. The patient stated that she had been gaining weight because she was terribly hungry all the time. She stated that she could not stay on her diet, but she had eliminated her feeding at bedtime. Poor control of diabetes followed this pattern: When the patient went to bed in the evening, urine sugar and acetone were negative. Upon rising the next morning, the patient had 4+ urine sugar with large amounts of acetone on numerous occasions. She stated that she frequently had nightmares and would awaken with her clothing saturated with perspiration.

On physical examination, the patient's height was 155 cm; her weight was 65 kg. The patient was normotensive and showed no signs of diabetic neuropathy or retinopathy.

Laboratory studies showed that on the same regimen the patient followed at home, fasting blood sugar was 520 mg/dl. Quantitative urine sugars during the day showed less than 4 gm of glucose; however, from 12 P.M. to 6 A.M., she spilled 22 gm sugar in the urine. Blood sugar drawn at 2 A.M. was 40 mg/dl; sugars drawn at 7 A.M. were frequently between 400 and 500 mg/dl.

Hospital course: The patient was placed on a 1,500 kcal American Diabetes Association (ADA) diet, which included a feeding at bedtime. Insulin dosage was gradually reduced, until the patient was taking 35 units NPH with 10 units regular insulin in the morning and 5 units NPH in the evening before supper. With this management, fasting blood sugars ranged from 150 to 200 mg/dl and 2-hour postprandial sugars ranged from 150 to 200 mg/dl; she spilled less than 20 gm sugar in the urine in 24 hours. The patient was quite active as an outpatient and was discharged on this same management. The patient was followed over the next several months. Her weight gradually fell by 4 kg, and the diabetes remained under good control.

Comment: This patient illustrates the Somogyi effect, i.e., posthypoglycemic hyperglycemia due to the administration of too much insulin. The clues to this condition were the patient's weight gain and the quick progression from negative urine sugar and acetone to 4+ urine sugar and acetone. The patient had made a bad choice when she discontinued her evening snack. This caused her to become hypoglycemic during the night. Hypoglycemia was manifested by nightmares and increased perspiration. She was overweight and needed a moderate degree of caloric restriction, with a concomitant reduction in insulin dosage.

It is now well established that obese patients are relatively resistant to insulin, whether endogenous or exogenous in origin.[26, 29, 41] The achievement of ideal body weight is therefore the most important therapeutic goal for both the insulin-dependent and the non-insulin-dependent diabetic. Adjustment of total caloric intake to obtain ideal body weight is the most important single factor to consider in prescribing the diet for a diabetic patient. It is also important that the number of calories ingested at a given time of day be constant from day to day to obtain a balance between the time of administration of insulin and exercise and the intake of calories.

The problems of the underweight, young diabetic patient are unique. It is exceedingly important to provide an adequate number of calories for normal growth and development. The first priority for the young, underweight diabetic in the growth phase should be the provision of calories; the dosage of insulin should be adjusted to whatever is needed to attain normal growth and weight. Total caloric intake must be adapted to the specific needs of the individual. One must take into account not only basic caloric requirements but adjustment of caloric requirements for activity.

CASE PRESENTATION.—D. B. is a 13-year-old boy who was referred for treatment because of short stature. This patient has had diabetes mellitus since the age of 6. His parents stated that he has had excellent control of the disease. They insisted that he adhered to a very strict diet of approximately 1,500 kcal/day. This diet kept blood sugars between 100 and 180 mg/dl, and urine sugar was negative. He has been taking 20 units NPH in the morning and 10 units NPH in the afternoon. His parents stated that his growth and development appeared to be normal until the onset of diabetes, when his rate of growth decreased; he was generally smaller than the other boys in his class.

Physical examination disclosed a small, apparently poorly nourished young man who was quite thin. He showed no physical signs of diabetic retinopathy or neuropathy. His pubis-to-floor and pubis-to-crown measurements were normal in proportion. His height and weight were 150 cm and 38 kg, respectively.

Laboratory studies showed fasting blood sugar 150 mg/dl, 2-hour postprandial blood sugar 180 mg/dl. A 24-hour urine contained no sugar.

It was our feeling that this patient's failure to grow was related to the marked restriction of caloric intake. During hospitalization, the patient was instructed to eat as many calories as required to satisfy his appetite. Urine and blood sugars were monitored closely, and insulin dosage was adjusted to maintain reasonable control of the diabetes. Caloric intake was calculated to be around 3,000 kcal/day.

The patient was discharged from the hospital on a 3,000 kcal ADA diet, which included a feeding at bedtime, and was taking 40 units NPH with 10 units regular insulin in the morning and 10 units NPH before supper.

On this treatment and regimen, the patient's fasting blood sugar was maintained between 150 and 200 mg/dl, and spillage of glucose in urine was under 20 gm/day. The patient experienced rather marked growth over the next year: His height increased to 160 cm; and his weight, to 50 kg.

Comment: This case illustrates the common misconception that the prognosis is poor for adolescents who require more than 40 units insulin per day; therefore, the caloric intake is restricted so that blood sugar can be controlled on 40 units insulin daily. During the growth period, it is exceedingly important to supply the required number of calories and nutrients for growth and adjust the insulin dosage to maintain reasonable control of diabetes during the growth phase. The outcome for this patient is typical; while calories were severely restricted, the patient's growth was severely retarded. With the administration of an appropriate number of calories and insulin, the patient grew normally.

Diet is the mainstay of the management of diabetes. It is impossible to regulate blood sugar by the administration of insulin, or any other drug, unless the diet is constant. The ability to calculate a diabetic diet using the exchange system is essential for any medical professional who is responsible for management of patients with this disease. The first step in this calculation is to determine the calories required to meet energy requirements according to sex, age, height and ideal body weight (see Chapter 2). After determining the number of calories required, it is necessary to calculate the distribution of calories as carbohydrate, protein and fat. The average American diet contains 40–50% carbohydrate, 10–15% protein and 40–45% fat. Currently, the most common composition of the diabetic diet is 40% carbohydrate, 20% protein and 40% fat. In some circles, carbohydrate intake is being increased to 45%, and fat is being reduced to 35%.

Example: 2,000 kcal/day required

$$2,000 \times 40\% = 800 \text{ kcal carbohydrate}$$
$$2,000 \times 20\% = 400 \text{ kcal protein}$$
$$2,000 \times 40\% = 800 \text{ kcal fat}$$
$$\text{carbohydrate} = 4 \text{ kcal/gm}$$
$$\text{protein} = 4 \text{ kcal/gm}$$
$$\text{fat} = 9 \text{ kcal/gm}$$
$$800 \text{ kcal carbohydrate} \div 4 = 200 \text{ gm carbohydrate}$$
$$400 \text{ kcal protein} \div 4 = 100 \text{ gm protein}$$
$$800 \text{ kcal fat} \div 9 = 90 \text{ gm fat}$$

TABLE 4-1.—FOOD VALUES FOR CALCULATION OF DIABETIC DIETS

FOOD GROUP	AMOUNT	CARBOHYDRATE (GM)	PROTEIN (GM)	FAT (GM)	KCAL
Milk, whole	1 cup	12	8	10	170
Vegetable A	As desired	–	–	–	–
Vegetable B	½ cup	5	2	–	28
Fruit	Varies	10	–	–	40
Bread exchange	Varies	15	2	–	68
Meat exchange°	1 oz	–	7	5	73
Fat exchange	1 tsp	–	–	5	45

°Meat exchanges have been divided into high, medium and low fat. Average figures are given here.

Another simple rule of thumb for calculating a diabetic diet for adults is to allow 1 gm protein/kg body weight and equally distribute the remaining kcal as carbohydrate and fat.

Carbohydrate and caloric intake should be evenly spaced throughout the day, usually in three meals plus a bedtime snack. For some patients, it is necessary to prevent hypoglycemia by prescribing snacks to be eaten at the time of peak insulin effect. However, calories from these snacks should be subtracted from the total calories in other meals. In our experience, the diabetic exchange system is extremely valuable and allows the diabetic to learn to choose foods under any circumstances. In the diabetic exchange system, foods are grouped by similar composition, i.e., each item listed in a particular food group contains the same number of calories and equal amounts of carbohydrates, protein and fat. For example, in the fruit exchange list, any listed fruit supplies 10 gm carbohydrate. The food values for the diabetic diet calculation are listed in Table 4-1. Actual calculation of the diet into the number of servings of bread, meat, fat exchanges, etc., required to complete the prescribed diet can be done as follows:

A. Start with basic nutritive requirements
   Milk   1 pt for adults; 1 qt for children
   Meat, fish, poultry, eggs   4–5 oz
      and cheese
   Fruit, one citrus or tomato   2 servings
   Vegetables, one green or   2 servings
      yellow
   Whole-grain or enriched   To meet caloric needs
      cereal or bread
   Fat or oil   To meet caloric needs
B. Subtract the number of gm carbohydrate furnished by 2 cups milk, 3 servings fruit, and 1 B-group vegetable from the amount prescribed (200

gm) and divide the result by 15, the number of gm carbohydrate in one serving from the bread exchange list.
C. Determine the amount of meat in the diet by subtracting the number of gm protein supplied by milk, vegetables and bread exchanges from the amount prescribed (100 gm) and divide the remainder by 7, the amount of protein in each meat exchange.
D. Follow the same procedure regarding fat, except divide the result by 5, the number of gm fat in one serving.

The patient's diet must be tailored to his or her accustomed eating habits and life-style; that is, if a patient is accustomed to eating his major meal at noon, that pattern should be continued, and insulin administration should be adjusted to that timing. Following any prescribed diet requires self-discipline, especially in our food- and alcohol-oriented society. Patients should be given recipes that help add variety to their diet. Several recipe books are available from the American Diabetes Association. The patient with diabetes needs periodic advice and encouragement to remain dedicated to adhering to his diet.

Problems Related to Calcium and Vitamin D

Osteoporosis

One of the most common disorders related to calcium and vitamin D metabolism is osteoporosis. This disease is characterized by a decrease in total bone mass, with the bone resorption rate exceeding the bone formation rate. The structure and mineral content of osteoporotic bone are normal; large resorption cavities are found, but the bone that is present has a normal ratio of calcium to matrix. From a nutritional point of view, the most important factors related to the development of osteoporosis are calcium and phosphorus intake. The serum calcium level must be maintained within very narrow margins. If calcium is not provided in the diet, it must be mobilized from bone to maintain normal serum calcium. Whenever the serum calcium level falls, the parathyroid gland is stimulated to secrete more parathyroid hormone (PTH), which causes calcium from bone to enter extracellular fluid and raise the serum calcium level.

Recent studies by Recker et al. suggest that women over 35 years of age require 1.3 gm of calcium per day to maintain a zero calcium balance.[30] They demonstrated that with an average calcium intake of 668 mg/day, women between the ages of 35 and 50 had a negative calcium balance of approximately 32 mg/day. Over a period of 30 years, 350 gm of calcium would be lost. Considering that the skeleton of an average-size woman at age 20 contains about 1,500 gm of calcium, then over a 30-year period, she would lose about 24% of total skeletal calcium. Many dietary surveys have suggested that it is not uncommon for women to consume only around 400 mg calcium per day. Obviously, calcium loss is much greater for these individuals.

Several groups have investigated the possibility that osteoporosis results from a chronically calcium-deficient diet. Urist found that 68% of osteoporotic women were on a low or borderline low calcium diet, that is, less than 800 mg of calcium per day.[39a] Nordin's study of 92 patients with osteoporosis and 92 controls revealed that more than half the patients with osteoporosis had calcium intakes of less than 14 mg/kg/day, while only about one fifth of the controls had calcium intakes under this amount. The osteoporotic individuals tended to have lower intakes of calcium and higher urinary excretion of calcium than normal subjects.[28]

Lutwak has emphasized the role that phosphate plays in calcium homeostasis.[27] In 1960, the ratio of dietary calcium to phosphorus was 1:2.8, with milk the primary source of calcium. There are several other major dietary sources of calcium, including poultry, fish and meat, which provide much larger amounts of phosphorus. Significant changes in the American diet have occurred since 1960. Milk consumption has decreased, while meat consumption has increased. Along with this trend has been a marked increase in the consumption of soft drinks, which contain large amounts of phosphorus in the form of phosphoric acid. These dietary changes have caused an increase in phosphorus intake and a decrease in calcium intake; the calcium phosphorus ratio now approaches 1:4. This increased intake of phosphorus affects calcium homeostasis in several ways. First, calcium absorption may be somewhat impaired when large concentrations of phosphorus are ingested; in addition, an increase in the intake of phosphorus lowers the serum ionized calcium concentration.[17] This fall in the ionized serum calcium level stimulates the secretion of PTH and leads to secondary hyperparathyroidism. In animal studies, a decreased ionized serum calcium level has been shown to be accompanied by the development of osteoporosis.[23]

The therapeutic implications of these findings seem obvious. It is essential that patients maintain an adequate intake of calcium and vitamin D, since calcium absorption is under the control of vitamin D (see Chapter 3). If patients avoid dairy products, it is very likely that they are on a low calcium diet. It is important to assess the dietary intake of calcium and if it is found to be low, the patients should be encouraged to increase calcium intake or should be given a calcium supplement unless contraindicated by, for example, hypercalcemia or hypercalcuria.

Patients with malabsorption have a more complicated problem, which is discussed extensively in Chapter 3. We would like to emphasize here that about 30% of patients who have had gastric surgery are susceptible to metabolic bone disease. Either overt or subclinical osteomalacia is the significant component in approximately 25% of patients; osteoporosis is seen in the other 5%.[9]

Familial Vitamin D-Resistant Rickets with Hypophosphatemia

Familial vitamin D-resistant rickets with hypophosphatemia is a specific disorder characterized by heredity, hypophosphatemia associated with decreased renal tubular reabsorption of inorganic phosphate, rickets, osteomalacia (which is not responsive to physiologic amounts of vitamin D), diminished gastrointestinal absorption of calcium and a questionable abnormality in the metabolism of vitamin D. Therapy for this syndrome consists of vitamin D, calcium and phosphate administration. It has been previously noted that phosphate and vitamin D supplements tend to lead to fewer cases of vitamin D intoxication.[37] It has been shown that ingestion of 1–3 gm of phosphorus per day in a neutral phosphate solution may in itself initiate and sustain healing for a certain period of time. In more prolonged observation of patients given phosphate alone, however, healing does not continue or may regress. Neutral phosphate solution containing 200–500 mg of phosphorus is usually given four times a day. Commercial preparations are available; for example, Fleet Phosphasoda contains 129 mg of phosphorus/ml. A neutral solution can be prepared by a pharmacist from mixtures of sodium or potassium mono- and dihydrogen phosphate in 4:1 molar ratio to obtain a pH of approximately 7.4. An important consideration in phosphate therapy is to dilute the phosphate in a sufficient amount of water to reduce osmolarity so that osmolar diarrhea will not be produced. The initial dose of vitamin D should be 10,000–25,000 u/day. The patient should then be seen at two-month intervals to measure serum calcium, phosphorus and alkaline phosphatase levels. The dosage of vitamin D can be increased in increments of 10,000 u/day every two months until the serum alkaline phosphatase level falls and serum phosphorus rises. When the alkaline phosphatase level begins to fall, the dosage of vitamin D should not be increased, and the patient should be carefully observed for signs of vitamin D intoxication. It must be emphasized

TABLE 4-2.—CALCIUM PREPARATION

Calcium gluconate 10 gm	= 1 gm calcium
Calcium lactate 8 gm	= 1 gm calcium
Calcium carbonate 2.5 gm	= 1 gm calcium

that any time vitamin D is given in pharmacologic doses, the serum calcium level must be followed at least every two months to prevent hypercalcemia. Calcium supplementation is usually given to provide 1 gm of elemental calcium daily in the form of calcium carbonate, lactate or gluconate. Elemental calcium content of each of these preparations is shown in Table 4-2.

Hypercalcemia

Dietary management of hypercalcemia is successful only for those syndromes in which hypercalcemia is due primarily to an increased intestinal absorption of calcium; i.e., vitamin D intoxication and sarcoidosis. For individuals with these syndromes, it is helpful to restrict calcium intake rather severely to levels between 150 to 400 mg/day. Phosphate is sometimes administered to control hypercalcemia and effectively lowers serum calcium; however, the complication of extraosseous calcification limits the usefulness of phosphate for treatment of these syndromes.

Calcium and Kidney Stones

This subject is discussed more fully in Chapter 7 on Nutrition and Diet Therapy in Renal Disease. The effectiveness of any therapy, whether diet or drug therapy, is very difficult to evaluate with accuracy. Howard and Thomas suggest that a patient probably should be followed for seven years before making any definite statements about the decrease or increase in incidence of stone formation by a given regimen.[19]

Diseases Manifest as Abnormalities in Metal Metabolism

WILSON'S DISEASE. — Wilson's disease is a rare, autosomal, recessively inherited disease characterized by degenerative changes in the brain, particularly the basal ganglia, and cirrhosis of the liver. Increased copper content in the liver and the brain has been demonstrated in Wilson's disease. Patients with Wilson's disease also have a diminished serum ceruloplasmin level. The relationship of the low ceruloplasmin level and the high tissue content of copper has not been well elucidated. Since treatment of Wilson's disease is designed to reduce the tissue store of copper, the copper content in the diet should be kept as low as possible. It is not possible to decrease the copper intake below 1 mg/day without severe caloric restriction; however, patients should be instructed to avoid high copper-containing foods, such as liver, nuts, mushrooms, chocolate and certain shell fish. Ingestion of potassium sulfide with meals has been advocated to reduce copper absorption. Effort also should be made to achieve an increase in the urinary excretion of copper. Agents that chelate copper have been used with some success. Dimercaprol (BAL) has been shown to increase urinary excretion, but it has some undesirable side effects. Penicillamine has proved very useful in the treatment of Wilson's disease. Its effect as a cupruretic agent is greater than that of BAL; its administration causes fewer adverse side effects. Its other advantage is that it can be given orally. This combination of decreased dietary intake of copper, combined with an increase in the urinary excretion, causes tissue depletion of copper.

HEMOCHROMATOSIS. — Primary hemochromatosis is characterized by the triad of cirrhosis, darkening of the skin and diabetes. The tissue content of iron is increased, and treatment is aimed at removing excess iron stores. As far as dietary management is concerned, it is obvious that these patients should not consume foods heavily fortified with iron.

Dietary Treatment of Inborn Errors of Metabolism

Inborn errors of metabolism result from absent or defective enzymes. As a result, there is an accumulation in the serum of the substrate upon which the deficient enzyme should act. In general, dietary management consists of limiting the intake of the substrate to prevent accumulation to toxic levels.

Since the theoretical possibility exists that there could be a defect in every step of the metabolic pathways, it would be impossible to discuss the management of each inborn error of metabolism. We will, therefore, limit ourselves to those defects most commonly encountered.

Inborn Errors of Amino Acid Metabolism

The inborn error of amino acid metabolism that has received the most attention is phenylketonuria. In this disorder, there is a defect in the hydroxylation of phenylalanine to tyrosine, which, if untreated, results in mental retardation.[25] The classical approach to treatment has been to reduce phenylalanine intake to levels sufficient enough to meet requirements for growth and tissue repair.[6] It is very difficult to strike the balance of limiting phenylalanine intake to prevent high accumulations of phenylalanine yet avoiding the consequences of phenylalanine deficiency; i.e., growth failure, anemia, generalized amino aciduria, hypoproteinemia and dermatitis.[18] It is mandatory that all essential amino acids be provided. In order to do this, low phenylalanine protein substitutes have been made commercially available. The most readily available preparation is Lofenalac. A teaspoonful of this supplement supplies 1.4 gm of protein and 7.5 mg phenylalanine. Phenylalanine from natural food sources and from Lofenalac supplies the total phenylalanine requirement of 70–90 mg/kg at one month of age, 35 mg/kg by 2 years, and 25 mg/kg at 10 years. The total phenylalanine content of milk in various formulas is listed in Table 4–3.

Although the relationship between the inactive phenylalanine hydroxylase enzyme and the mental retardation which inevitably ensues with untreated phenylketonuria is not understood, we do know that when phenylalanine is reduced, a child can develop normally.[15] Treatment must begin as early in infancy as possible. Kang et al. found that the mean intelligence quotient (IQ) of 27 patients with phenylketonuria treated before three weeks of age was comparable to the IQ of unaffected siblings. However, the mean IQ of 12 patients treated between three and six weeks of age was significantly below the mean IQ of their unaffected siblings.[24] It should be pointed out, however, that improvement in mental function has been reported in patients who have been treated as late as 2 or 3 years of age.[13] A collaborative study of children with phenylketonuria suggested that there was no significant difference in IQ or in performance between groups of children whose phenylalanine levels were maintained between 5.5 and 9.9 mg/dl.[42] As a result of this study, clinicians have become less strict in their dietary restrictions. Most clinicians feel that results are acceptable if the serum phenylalanine levels are kept between 4 and 10 mg dl.

TABLE 4–3.—PHENYLALANINE
CONTENT OF MILK

MILK	DILUTION	PHENYLALANINE (MG/OZ)
Cow	–	51
Similac	1:1	27
Human	–	19
Lofenalac	1:2	3.5

The discussion thus far has been directed at patients with classical phenylketonuria. Atypical phenylketonuria or hyperphenylalanemia is due to a *reduction* in phenylalanine hydroxylase, but the enzyme is present. Infants with hyperphenylalanemia usually do not have severe neurologic damage. There is some question whether dietary management of these individuals is necessary, except when it is indicated during pregnancy.[6]

Maple syrup urine disease, or branched-chain hyperaminoacidemia, is due to an enzyme defect involving the degradation of leucine, isoleucine and valine and an accumulation of metabolites proximal to the metabolic block. Treatment involves the avoidance of excesses of these three essential amino acids by supplying purified amino acids and natural food supplements to maintain growth. Early introduction and maintenance of the diet helps to avoid neurologic problems.[43]

Homocystinuria is due to a deficiency in cystathionine synthetase, which converts homocystine and serine to cystathionine, and results in an accumulation of homocystine and methionine in the blood and urine.[6, 18] Requirements for exogenous cystine are increased in homocystinuria. On the other hand, dietary methionine should be restricted to lower the plasma methionine and homocystine levels. Special low methionine diets should be supplemented with cystine and cysteine, folate and choline. In some instances, pyridoxine in dosages of 150–1,200 mg/day can reduce serum homocystine levels.

Porphyria is thought to be due to an increase in the activity of liver δ aminolevulinic acid (ALA) synthetase, which may be due to faulty feedback inhibition of the enzyme. Porphyria results in the excretion in the urine of large amounts of ALA, porphobilinogen (PBG) and porphyrins. Increased carbohydrate intake appears to be associated with decreased PBG excretion.[18]

Cystinosis is a metabolic disorder biochemically characterized by high intracellular content of free cystine, which results in crystal deposits in the cornea, kidney, bone marrow, lymph nodes, leukocytes and liver. Cystinosis has a wide range of clinical expression. In the most severe form of the disease, crystal deposits in the kidney cause generalized renal tubular dysfunction and progressive renal damage. In some cases, cystinosis is discovered serendipitously by an opthalmologist, who discovers crystals in the cornea and conjunctivae. Experimental treatment with a diet restricted in cystine and methionine and administration of penicillamine, which chelates cystine and methionine, failed to influence the course of the disease.[4]

Cystinuria is due to a hereditary abnormality of transport in which the intestinal absorption and renal tubular reabsorption of cystine, lysine, arginine and ornithine is impaired. These amino acids are then excreted in the urine in abnormally high amounts throughout life. The major complication of this disorder is the formation of cystine stones. A high concentration of cystine in the urine near solubility limit produces stones by precipitation. Treatment of stones is aimed at lowering the total amount of cystine in the urine, lowering the concentration of cystine by increasing the volume of urine or increasing the solubility of cystine in the urine. The amount of cystine in the urine is a reflection of its level in the blood, and it is difficult to control. It is replenished from tissue sources and dietary precursors, principally methionine. The avoidance of excess intake of protein, especially from animal sources that are high in methionine, can significantly limit the amount of cystine excreted. Increase in urine volume by the administration of large amounts of fluid is extremely important in the management of patients with cystinuria. Dent recommended diuresis to avoid supersaturated urine in early morning.[8] In addition to high daytime water intake (500 ml every four hours), patients were instructed to drink two glasses of water at bedtime and two glasses at 2 A.M. Periodic tests of cystine concentration in morning urine showed that at no time was supersaturated urine found, nor was there deposition of stones. Since cystine is much more soluble in alkaline media, increasing the pH of the urine is also beneficial. Alkalinization of the urine can be aided by ingestion of a high vegetable (except corn and lentils), high fruit (excluding cranberries, plums and prunes) diet. However, this diet is not adequate to achieve a pH of 7.5, the maximum alkalinity at which cystine solubility is increased; therefore, alkali therapy, such as potassium bicarbonate or citrate, must be added.

Inborn Errors of Carbohydrate Metabolism

Galactosemia is due to deficiency of galactokinase or galacto-1-phosphate uridyl transferase, which results in an increased tissue content of galactose. Treatment consists of withdrawal of galactose through a low galactose diet or galactose-free formula for infants. Peas, lima beans, sugar beets, liver, pancreas and brains should be avoided.[18]

Lactase deficiency has been discussed at some length in Chapter 3.

Fructosemia results from a deficiency of fructose-1-phosphate aldolase, causing accumulation of fructose-1-phosphate in the liver and slow clearing of fructose from the serum.[6, 18] Treatment consists of fructose-free diets, as well as the elimination of foods containing sucrose. Vegetables and many fruits supply an ascorbic acid-containing sucrose; so it is necessary to replace vitamin C by sucrose-free, artificial vitamin C preparations.

Sucrose 1-1 isomaltase deficiency results in an inability to break down the branch starches, or amylopectins, contained in potatoes and wheat; therefore, these foods should be avoided. Sucrose must be avoided as well. It has been possible to manage this disorder satisfactorily by using fungal sucrose preparations without dietary restriction of the substrates.

REFERENCES

1. Berman, J. L.: Phenylketonuria, Am. Fam. Physician 3:113, 1971.
2. Berry, H. K., Hunt, M. M., and Sutherland, B. K.: Amino acid balance in the treatment of phenylketonuria, J. Am. Diet. Assoc. 58:210, 1971.
3. Brunzell, J. D., et al.: Improved glucose tolerance with high carbohydrate feeding in mild diabetes, New Engl. J. Med. 284:521, 1971.
4. Christensen, M. D., Nielsen, J. A., and Henriksen, O.: Treatment of cystinosis with a diet poor in cystine and methionine, Acta Paediatr. Scand. 59:613, 1970.
5. Committee on Food and Nutrition, American Diabetes Association: Principles of nutrition and dietary recommendations for patients with diabetes mellitus, Diabetes 20:633, 1971.
6. Dancis, J.: Nutritional management of hereditary disorders, Med. Clin. North Am. 54:1431, 1970.
7. Demanet, J. C., and Vryens, R.: Advantage of a high sodium diet in the diagnosis of hyperaldosteronism, Horm. Metab. Res. 3:442, 1971.
8. Dent, C. E., and Senior, B.: Studies in the treatment of cystinuria, Br. J. Urol, 27:317, 1955.
9. Eddy, R. L.: Metabolic bone disease after gastrectomy, Am. J. Med. 50: 442, 1971.
10. Fisch, R. O., et al.: Twelve years of clinical experience with phenylketonuria, Neurology (Minneap.), 19:659, 1969.
11. Gershon-Cohen, J., and Jowsey, J.: The relationship of dietary calcium to osteoporosis, Metabolism 13:221, 1964.
12. Hales, C. N.: The role of insulin in the regulation of glucose metabolism, Proc. Nutr. Soc. 30:282, 1971.
13. Hambraeus, L., Holmgren, G., and Samuelson, G.: Dietary treatment of adult patients with phenylketonuria, Nutr. Metab. 13:298, 1971.
14. Hambraeus, L., Wranne, L., and Lorentsson, R.: Whey protein formulas in the treatment of phenylketonuria in infants, Nutr. Metab. 12:152, 1970
15. Hanley, W. B., Linsao, L. S., and Netley, C.: The efficacy of dietary therapy for phenylketonuria, Can. Med. Assoc. J. 104:1089, 1971.
16. Harries, J. T., et al.: Low proline diet in type I hyperprolinaemia, Arch. Dis. Child. 46:72, 1971.
17. Herbert, L. A., Lemann, J. J., Peterson, J. R.: Studies of the mechanism by which phosphate infusion lowers serum calcium concentration, J. Clin. Invest. 45:1886, 1966.
18. Holtzman, N. A.: Dietary treatment of inborn errors of metabolism, Annu. Rev. Med. 21:335, 1970.
19. Howard, J. E., and Thomas W. C.: Control of crystallization in urine, Am. J. Med. 45:693, 1968.
20. Hunt, M. M., Sutherland, B. S., and Berry, H. K.: Nutritional management in phenylketonuria, Am. J. Dis. Child. 122:1, 1971.

21. Jackson, R. L.: The child with diabetes, Nutr. Today, 6:2, 1971.
22. Jenkins, D. J. A., et al.: Unabsorbable carbohydrates and diabetes: Decreased postprandial hyperglycemia, Lancet 2:172, 1976.
23. Jowsey, J., Reiss, E., Canterbury, J. M.: Long-term effects of high phosphate intake on parathyroid hormone levels and bone metabolism, Acta Orthop. Scand. 45:801, 1974.
24. Kang, E. S., Sollee, N. D., and Gerald, P. S.: Results of treatment and termination of the diet in phenylketonuria (PKU), Pediatrics 46:881, 1970.
25. Knox, W. E.: Phenylketonuria, in Stanbury, J. B., Wyngaarden, J. B., and Fredrickson, D. S. (eds.): The Metabolic Basis of Inherited Disease (3d ed.; New York: McGraw-Hill Book Company, 1972), pp. 266–295.
26. Kreisberg, R. A., Owen, W. C., and Siegal, A. M.: Nutrition and endocrine disease, Med. Clin. North Am. 54:1473, 1970.
27. Lutwak, L., et al.: J. Med. Sci. 7:504, 1971.
28. Nordin, B. E. C.: Osteoporosis and calcium deficiency, in Rodahl, K., Nicholson, J. T., and Brown, E. M. (eds.): Bone as a Tissue (New York: McGraw-Hill Book Company, 1960), p. 46.
29. Rabinowitz, D., Zierler, K. L.: Forearm metabolism in obesity and its response to intra-arterial insulin. Characterization of insulin resistance and evidence for adaptive hyperinsulinism, J. Clin. Invest. 41:2173, 1962.
30. Recker, R. R., Saville, P. D., and Heaney, R. P.: Sex hormones or calcium supplements diminish postmenopausal bone loss, Clin. Res. 24:583A, 1976.
31. Sharkey, T. P.: Diabetes mellitus—present problems and new research, I–III. Prevalence in the United States, J. Am. Diet. Assoc. 58:201, 1971.
32. Sharkey, T. P.: Diabetes mellitus—present problems and new research, IV, V. The heart and vascular disease, J. Am. Diet. Assoc. 58:336, 1971.
33. Sharkey, T. P.: Diabetes mellitus—present problems and new research, VI. Retinopathy and neuropathy, J. Am. Diet. Assoc. 58:441, 1971.
34. Sharkey, T. P.: Diabetes mellitus—present problems and new research, VII. Retinopathy, J. Am. Diet. Assoc. 58:528, 1971.
35. Sharkey, T. P.: Sorbitol and mannitol for diabetic patients, J. Am. Diet. Assoc. 58:570, 1971.
36. Shih, V. E.: Early dietary management in an infant with arginosuccinase deficiency: Preliminary report, J. Pediatr. 80:645, 1972.
37. Stickler, G. B., Hayles, A. B., and Rosevarju: Familial hypophosphatemic, vitamin D-resistant rickets: Effect of increased oral calcium and phosphorus intake without high doses of vitamin D, Am. J. Dis. Child. 110:664, 1975.
38. Sutherland, B. S., Berry, H. K., and Umbarger, B.: Growth and nutrition in treated phenylketonuria patients, J.A.M.A. 211:270, 1970.
39. Szabo, O., and Mahler, R. J.: The influence of fatty acid ingestion upon oral glucose tolerance, Horm. Metab. Res. 3:299, 1971.
39a. Urist, M. R., Gurvey, M. S., and Fareed, D. O.: Long-term Observations on Aged Women with Pathologic Osteoporosis, in Garzel, U. S. (ed.): Osteoporosis (New York: Grune & Stratton, Inc., 1969), pp. 3–37.
40. Watkins, M. L., Crump, E. P., and Hara, S.: Management of transient hyperphenylalaninemia and tyrosinemia in low birth weight Negro infants fed high protein diets, J. Natl. Med. Assoc. 63:241, 1971.

41. West, K. M., and Kalbfleisch, J. M.: Influence of nutritional factors on prevalence of diabetes, Diabetes 20:99, 1971.
42. Williamson, M., Koch, R., and Dolson, J. C.: Phenylketonuria collaborative study current status. A report presented at the 3rd I.A.F.F.M.D. Congress, The Hague, The Netherlands, 1973.
43. Wong, P. W. K., et al.: A case of classical maple syrup urine disease: Thiamine nonresponsive, Clin. Genet. 3:27, 1972.
44. Wood, F. C., and Bierman, E. L.: New concepts in diabetic dietetics, Nutr. Today 7:4, 1972.
45. Yu, J. S., Stuckey, S. J., and O'Halloran, M. T.: Atypical phenylketonuria: An approach to diagnosis and management, Arch. Dis. Child. 45:561, 1970.
46. Yu, J. S., Stuckey, S. J., and O'Halloran, M. T.: The dangers of dietary therapy in phenylketonuria, Med. J. Aust. 2:404, 1970.

Chapter 5 / Nutrition in Cardiovascular Disease

THE IMPORTANCE of nutrition in the management of cardiovascular disease is well recognized but frequently not emphasized.

Before the availability of thiazide diuretics, sodium restriction was the backbone of therapy for both congestive heart failure and hypertension. With the availability of potent diuretics, some physicians began to underemphasize the importance of the low sodium diet. This is unfortunate, since a continued high sodium intake not only tends to negate the beneficial effect of diuretics but also accentuates electrolyte disturbances, particularly hypokalemia, produced by diuretics.

The role of dietary intake of saturated fat in the pathogenesis of atherosclerosis is under scrutiny. The mechanisms by which a decrease in dietary saturated fat and an increase in dietary polyunsaturated fat alters serum cholesterol are controversial.[32] However, the Oslo Heart study suggests that limitation of dietary saturated fat may be beneficial.[19]

This chapter will deal with the role of diet and dietary management in the treatment of diseases of the cardiovascular system.

Hypertension

Hypertension is a common abnormality produced by a variety of disease processes. It also causes a number of serious disorders, ranging from cardiac muscle hypertrophy to myocardial infarction and cerebral hemorrhage. Essential hypertension is by far the most common form of hypertensive disease, and it is the only form that will be dealt with here. In essential hypertension, diffuse constriction of the arterioles causes elevation of the arterial pressure.

Expansion of blood volume due to sodium retention may play a role in hypertension. According to Tobian, hypertensive patients have an excessive amount of sodium in the walls of their arteries, which causes an increase in the sensitivity of the arterioles to the constrictive effect of catecholamines.[38] By restricting dietary sodium, total body sodium and water are decreased, thus decreasing circulating blood volume and sodium content in the arterioles.

There is epidemiologic evidence available that suggests that there may be some correlation between salt intake and hypertension in

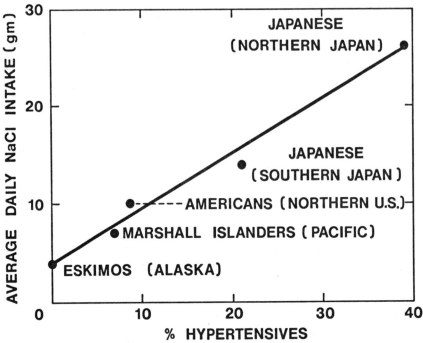

Fig 5–1.—Relationship between dietary intake of salt and the incidence of hypertension. (From Dahl, L. K.: Salt Intake in the Development of Essential Hypertension, in *Essential Hypertension,* International CIBA Symposium [Heidelberg: Springer Verlag, 1960]. Used by permission.)

man. Surveys of geographical areas published by Dahl in 1960 show a positive correlation between the daily salt intake and hypertension (Fig 5–1).

Obesity is a common companion of hypertension. Some investigators feel that obese patients with certain personality types tend to be prone to essential hypertension. In addition, the obese patient usually has an expanded extracellular fluid volume and an increased capillary bed size, both of which tend to elevate the blood pressure.

CASE PRESENTATION.—M. H. is a 53-year-old woman who was seen for a general physical evaluation. Her only complaints were steady weight gain and occasional occipital headache upon awakening.

Physical examination revealed an obese woman. Her height was 139.7 cm, weight 95.4 kg. The fundi showed grade II hypertensive retinopathy. Heart rate was 88 beats/min; no murmurs were found. Blood pressure was 180/110 mm Hg; chest was clear; abdomen was negative. There was 1+ edema of the ankles.

Laboratory work disclosed that CBC, UA, BUN, creatinine, electrolytes, 24-

hour urine vanillylmandelic acid (VMA) and hypertensive intravenous pyelogram (IVP) were normal.

The patient was placed on a 1,500 mg sodium and 1,200 cal diet. After three weeks, she had lost 3.6 kg, and her blood pressure was 170/100 mm Hg. Added to her management were 50 mg hydrochlorothiazide daily and 20 mEq/L potassium chloride twice a day. After one year, the patient weighed 68.2 kg, and her blood pressure was 140/80 mm Hg. At this point, it was decided to discontinue administration of the thiazide diuretic and potassium chloride. The patient's blood pressure was then maintained at 140/80 mm Hg by diet alone.

DIETARY CONSIDERATIONS.—Restriction of calories helps prevent great fluctuations in blood pressure after the ingestion of large meals. Such fluctuations in blood pressure are due to decreased efficiency of vasomotor regulation in patients with essential hypertension. In the obese patient, the heart labors under a double load from hypertension and excess body weight. For rapid weight loss in a severely hypertensive patient, a caloric restriction of 1,000 to 1,200 kcal/day is recommended.[16] For this patient, a 1,200-kcal diet was established.

Sodium restriction augments the effectiveness of such drugs as ganglionic blocking agents, adrenergic blockers or competitive inhibitors of catecholamine vasoconstrictors. Years ago, dietary treatment consisted of only 200 mg sodium per day. Kempner's Rice-Fruit Diet in 1944 contained no animal protein and led to negative nitrogen balance. At present, the sodium restriction may vary, depending on the severity of hypertension. Usually, restrictions range from 500 to 3,000 mg sodium per day; 1,500 mg sodium is a more realistic restriction for severely hypertensive patients to follow at home.

Excess dietary sodium has been shown to induce hypertension in rats and to increase its severity in humans with a family history of hypertension. Dahl has recommended that human salt intake be no greater than 5 gm per day, which is 2,000 mg sodium (40% of salt is sodium).[10] The average American diet contains approximately 6,000 mg sodium per day. The advice, "just cut down on sodium intake," is nearly useless in most cases. Patients tend to equate sodium *only* with visible salt in the salt shaker and do not understand that sodium is naturally present in all foods. Jean Mayer outlined rules that pertain to a mildly restricted, low sodium diet and to a severe sodium restriction.[25, 26] However, some of his suggestions were too liberal for a 1,500 mg sodium diet. All foods and beverages contain some sodium naturally. Therefore, it is necessary to be more specific when counseling a patient about his sodium restriction. Below is a list of items that contain sodium and are often not eliminated by the patient who requires sodium restriction:

Accent (monosodium glutamate) Meat tenderizer
Soy sauce Softened water
Baking soda Some sugar substitutes
Commercially prepared foods Preservatives
Dietetic soft drinks Mold inhibitors
Canned vegetables Certain medicines and dentifrices

Patients should be instructed to read *all* labels on food, and to look for the words "soda" and "sodium" or the symbol "Na," all of which should be avoided.

The advice and guidance of a dietitian is also necessary for each patient so that the diet can be "tailored" to the patient's way of life as much as possible. Helpful seasoning and cooking suggestions from the dietitian are needed if the patient is expected to adhere to a diet with so many restrictions and low sodium products. Sodium values for several foods that frequently present problems are given in Table 5-1.

TABLE 5-1.—SODIUM VALUES OF
SOME FOODS

FOODS	NA VALUE (MG)
1 slice bacon	76
1 cup buttermilk	215
1 tbsp catsup	177
1 oz cheddar cheese	420
2 in. square cornbread	283
1 cup dialyzed milk	7
1 egg	65
1 oz meat, fish, poultry	25
1 cup milk	122
1 tsp butter or margarine	49
1 saltine cracker	35
1 tbsp mayonnaise	84
1 slice rye bread	128
1 slice white bread	117
3 oz shrimp	120
¼ tsp sodium chloride	600
1 slice low-sodium bread	6
1 cup canned tomato juice	500
½ cup seasoned carrots, spinach or beets	200
½ cup sauerkraut	500
1 oz canned tuna	200
5 salted nuts	200
½ cup raw carrots or celery	50

1 mEq Na = 23 mg
1,500 mg Na = approximately 65 mEq

Congestive Heart Failure

Abnormal retention of sodium and water is one of the earliest findings in chronic congestive heart failure. As a result, the extracellular fluid expands, predisposing the patient to edema and increasing the load on the heart by increasing venous return. The cause of abnormal sodium retention in early congestive heart failure remains unsettled. Renin levels are increased, and the aldosterone secretion rate is elevated in some patients with congestive heart failure. This is probably secondary to a decrease in perfusion pressure in afferent arterioles to the juxtaglomerular apparatus in the kidney. In bilaterally adrenalectomized animals maintained on constant doses of deoxycorticosterone, salt retention occurs when the heart fails. However, mineralocorticoids are metabolized at an abnormally slow rate in patients with heart failure, and the plasma aldosterone level is often high, even when the secretion rate is normal. Other possible mechanisms for sodium retention have been suggested.

CASE PRESENTATION.—I. S. is a 71-year-old woman who was admitted to the hospital with the chief complaints of shortness of breath and swelling of the ankles. These symptoms had become progressively worse over the past month. The patient had a long history of hypertension.

Physical examination revealed an obese, elderly woman who was acutely short of breath. Her height was 170 cm, weight 81 kg. Heart rate was 120 beats/min; and summation gallop was detected. Blood pressure was 180/100 mm Hg. There was dullness to percussion over the lower half of the chest, diminished breath sounds and rales bilaterally. There was abdominal ascites, and the liver was palpable 7 cm below the right costal margin. There was 4+ pitting edema of the knees.

During hospitalization, the patient responded well to bed rest, digitalization, sodium restriction and diuretics. She lost 13.5 kg during diuresis.

The patient was discharged on 0.25 mg digoxin daily, 25 mg spironolactone (Aldactone) four times a day, 40 mg furosemide (Lasix) daily and a 1,000 cal, 1,500 mg sodium diet. She did well for several weeks. When the patient was seen in the outpatient clinic on two occasions, her weight remained stable, and cardiac status remained compensated. However, on her third clinic visit, she had gained 8 kg in a three-week period despite taking the same medications. She was in obvious heart failure. When taking a history, it was found that the patient had been eating Kentucky Fried Chicken daily, which greatly increased her sodium intake.

DIETARY CONSIDERATIONS.—If a patient is obese, weight reduction is a must. Obesity increases the work of the heart during exertion and is a handicap to circulation and respiration. Past dietary treatment ranged from Karells' diet in 1866, which consisted of only 800 ml milk per day, to Acid-Ash diets to enhance mercurial diuresis, to reduction diets of 800–1,200 kcal and 60–70 gm protein. Starvation has been used in the past as part of the treatment of congestive heart failure. Success with this form of treatment is based on the marked sodium and water diuresis that accompanies the ketosis of starvation.[8] Present dietary treatment emphasizes a kcal level to reach and maintain "ideal" weight for the patient's height and age. For this patient, a 1,000 kcal diet was established.

Sodium restriction is necessary, especially if the kidneys are unable to excrete salt and water adequately because of impaired renal hemodynamics and hormonal factors from inadequate cardiac output. For the cardiac patient with refractory congestive heart failure, a 500 mg sodium diet is suggested. However, for many patients, a restriction to 1,500–2,000 mg sodium per day will suffice.

Potassium may be depleted as a consequence of chronic therapy with diuretics, whose action in the nephron is proximal to the potassium-hydrogen exchange site. With submaximal doses of thiazides for hypertension or with intermittent use of diuretics for mild congestive heart failure, it is often suggested that potassium depletion can be countered by ensuring an adequate amount of potassium in the diet, especially in the form of fruit or fruit juices. Bateson and Lant found that only 3 of 100 ward patients were drinking real fruit juice with a potassium content of 25 mEq/500 ml.[5] Most of the proprietary drinks had a maximum content of potassium equal to 8.9 mEq/L. Normal dai-

TABLE 5–2.—POTASSIUM-
RICH FOODS°

FOODS	K VALUE (MG)
1 cup whole milk	356
1 cup grapefruit juice	405
1 cup orange juice	496
1 cup canned tomato juice	536
½ cup lima beans	352
1 oz beet greens	570
1 oz bitter chocolate	235
1 oz plain cocoa	432
1 small banana	420
10 medium dates	648
1 tbsp peanut butter	246
½ cup raw potatoes	407

°Potassium content of foods is affected by geographic, climatic, and processing factors.
1 mEq K = 39 mg.

ly intake is 40–100 mEq potassium. In order to increase this intake by an additional 25 mEq, an intake of 500 ml or even more real fruit juice is necessary. Potassium supplements are recommended to make up the potassium deficit, since supplements are usually less expensive and are a sure and easy way to meet a patient's increased potassium requirement. A list of the potassium content of some "potassium-rich" foods is shown in Table 5–2.

Dietary Treatment for Acute Myocardial Infarction

For the first two to three days after acute myocardial infarction, a liquid diet of 1,000–1,500 ml/day should be given. Liquids should be restricted in sodium to prevent further complications and a rise in blood pressure. As soon as the patient can tolerate soft foods, fluids should be supplemented by small portions of sodium-restricted cooked foods in multiple feedings to prevent further embarrassment to the heart. After the acute phase, a diet of 800–1,200 kcal can be initiated and gradually increased as the patient improves. If the patient is obese, his weight should be reduced to "ideal" weight for his height and age. Sodium intake should be regulated for patients who show signs of congestive heart failure or hypertension.

According to the Oslo Heart study, a diet low in saturated fats and cholesterol and high in polyunsaturated fats reduces the incidence of fatal and nonfatal myocardial reinfarction.[19] Further discussion of this type of diet appears in the section of this chapter on hyperlipoproteinemias

Serum Lipid Disorders and Atherosclerosis

According to Fredrickson, the five types of hyperlipoproteinemia are of significant importance in the diagnosis and treatment of various serum lipid disorders. Certain types of hyperlipidemia are associated with a high risk of premature atherosclerosis. Proper clinical management is achieved most effectively by translation of hyperlipidemia into hyperlipoproteinemia. The classification described in this text has been proposed by a select committee of the World Health Organization.[6]

It might be well to review serum lipids before progressing to the lipemias. Normal blood plasma in man contains about 500 mg total lipid/100 ml. Of the total lipid, 180 mg or more is cholesterol; $2/3$ is esterified with fatty acids, and $1/3$ is present as free sterol. Phosphoglycerides constitute about 160 mg; and about $1/4$ is triacylglycerol (tri-

TABLE 5-3.—LIPOPROTEINS OF HUMAN PLASMA

	FRACTION				
	CHYLOMICRONS	VERY LOW DENSITY	LOW DENSITY	HIGH DENSITY	VERY HIGH DENSITY
Density	<1.006	1.006–1.019	1.019–1.063	1.063–1.21	>1.21
S_f	>400	12–400	0–12	–	–
Diameter, Å	5,000–10,000	300–700	200–250	100–150	100
Electrophoretic fraction	$\alpha 2$	$\beta 1$	$\beta 1$	$\alpha 1$	$\alpha 1$
Amount, mg/100 ml plasma	100–250	130–200	210–400	50–130	290–400
Approximate percentage composition					
Protein	2	9	21	33	57
Phosphoglyceride	7	18	22	29	21
Cholesterol					
Free	2	7	8	7	3
Ester	6	15	38	23	14
Triacylglycerol	83	50	10	8	5
Fatty acids	–	1	1	–	–

From White, A., Handler, P., and Smith, E. L.: *Principles of Biochemistry* (5th ed.; New York: McGraw-Hill Book Company, 1973), p. 547

glycerides). Increase in the amount of serum lipid is termed *lipemia*. Lipoprotein fractions can be separated by repeated centrifugation of the plasma at high speeds and may be characterized by their flotation constants and the densities at which they separate. The fractions of lowest density are richest in triacylglycerols and poorest in protein. Determinations of the distribution or relative concentrations of the lipoprotein fractions or the lipids in these fractions are more informative than estimations of the total concentration of a specific lipid in plasma. Table 5–3 demonstrates the density of various lipoproteins in human plasma.

The most common and widely available method for lipoprotein analysis is electrophoresis. Using the difference in charge of the lipoprotein moieties, one may define a nonmigrating, a β-migrating, a pre-β-migrating and an α-migrating lipoprotein band. A drop of the patient's plasma on filter paper or agarose gel is put into an electrophoretic cell containing a buffer solution of albumin. The lipid-rich particles remaining at the origin correlate well with centrifugally defined chylomicrons, the β-lipoproteins with low-density lipoprotein (LDL), the pre-β-lipoproteins with very low-density lipoproteins (VLDL), and the α-lipoproteins with high-density lipoproteins (HDL).[20]

Decisions about dietary management are made on the basis of the type of hyperlipoproteinemia. It is important to remember that the serum lipid and lipoprotein pattern should be checked approximately six to eight weeks after altering the diet.

Type I Hyperlipoproteinemia (Hyperchylomicronemia)

This disease usually is seen in young patients who present with the complaint of frequent abdominal pain associated with ingestion of dietary fat. In addition to bouts of abdominal pain, patients may have lipemia retinalis, hepatosplenomegaly and eruptive xanthomas. Type I hyperlipoproteinemia is nearly always familial but may occasionally be secondary to dysglobulinemia or insulinopenic diabetes mellitus. Etiology of the familial disorder is thought to be a genetic deficiency of lipoprotein lipase, which is responsible for clearing chylomicrons from the plasma. There is no increased incidence of diabetes mellitus or atherosclerosis.

The type I lipoprotein pattern indicates an inability to clear chylomicrons. Plasma cholesterol may be normal or elevated; triglyceride levels are grossly elevated, often above 5,000 mg/dl. Plasma from these patients appears creamy; after standing in the cold, a discrete cream layer forms in the plasma.

Dietary treatment consists of a low-fat diet (25–35 gm per day). The rationale is as follows: Fats absorbed as fatty acids from long-chain triglycerides are reformed within the epithelial cell to triglycerides. Triglycerides combine with lipoprotein to form chylomicrons. Due to the deficiency of lipoprotein lipase in patients with type I hyperlipoproteinemia, the chylomicrons accumulate and result in a rise of serum triglycerides. Restricting fat in the diet minimizes chylomicron formation. Since protein foods, such as meat, contain fat as well, the protein allowance is restricted to 5 oz meat per day (1 oz lean meat is 8 gm protein and 3 gm fat). Butter, margarine, shortening, oils, nuts and baked goods are eliminated. Dairy products containing fat are restricted, and milk should be skim, not low fat or 2%. Medium-chain triglycerides (MCT) can be used in the diet, since they enter the blood stream directly as fatty acids after digestion and bypass the lymph system. Generally, cholesterol is not limited in the diet. Bread, cereals, vegetables (cooked plainly) and fruit are not limited. None of the presently available antilipemic drugs has shown any sustained effect on this exogenous hypertriglyceridemia.

Type IIa Hyperlipoproteinemia

CASE PRESENTATION.—W. S. is a 51-year-old man who presented with the chief complaint of sustained chest pain on exertion. Coronary arteriograms showed severe three-vessel arteriosclerotic disease, with 90% occlusion of the left anterior descending coronary artery.

Past medical history revealed that the patient had been asymptomatic, with no major illnesses in his life. However, he had had significant fluctuations in weight, with a tendency toward obesity. From early childhood, he had eaten a diet high in saturated fat. He was quite sedentary and did not enjoy exercise.

Family history revealed that his mother had suffered a myocardial infarction at age 58; a brother had a myocardial infarction at age 50; and a maternal uncle died from a "heart attack" at age 48.

Physical examination revealed an alert man who appeared to be his stated age. His height was 177.8 cm, weight 70.5 kg. There were no significant abnormalities.

Laboratory work revealed normal CBC, BUN, creatinine, 2-hour postprandial blood sugar, electrolytes and thyroxin. The serum lipoprotein electrophoresis showed a type IIa pattern, with 296 mg/dl cholesterol and 100 mg/dl triglycerides.

Subsequent serum lipoprotein electrophoresis was performed on six of his seven siblings. Three had type IIa patterns; two had type IV patterns; one had a normal pattern.

The patient was placed on a type IIa hyperlipoproteinemia diet. His

Fig 5–2.—Model showing absence of receptor sites for low-density lipoprotein *(LDL)* in patients with type IIa hyperlipoproteinemia. (From Goldstein, J. L., and Brown, M. S.: J. Lab. Clin. Med. 85:15, 1975. Used by permission.)

FAMILIAL HYPERCHOLESTEROLEMIA
MODEL FOR PATHOGENESIS

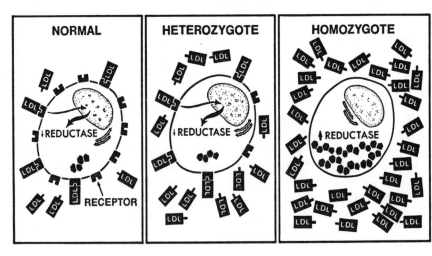

NORMAL | HETEROZYGOTE | HOMOZYGOTE

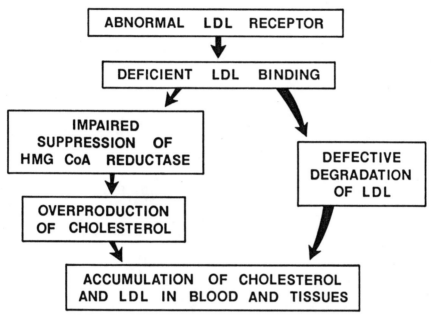

Fig 5–3.—Sequence of events in absence of receptors for low-density lipoprotein *(LDL)* in cells of patients with familial type IIa hypercholesterolemia. (From Goldstein, J. L., and Brown, M. S.: J. Lab. Clin. Med. 85:15, 1975. Used by permission.)

cholesterol fell to 240 mg/dl, and the type IIa pattern reverted to normal.

This patient demonstrated the most common morbidity of type IIa hyperlipoproteinemia; i.e., coronary artery disease. His unfavorable course was probably accelerated by genetic predisposition and a diet high in saturated fat.

Type IIa hyperlipoproteinemia is manifested by an increase in β-lipoprotein and cholesterol. It is a relatively common inheritable disorder. Goldstein has provided convincing evidence that patients with familial hypercholesterolemia have a defect in the cell surface receptor for LDL.[15] This appears to have two important consequences: (1) the cell cannot suppress activity of 3-hydroxy-3-methylglutaryl coenzyme A reductase (HMG CoA), the rate-limiting enzyme for cholesterologenesis in the liver; and (2) the cell cannot degrade LDL when it is present in low concentrations extracellularly. The consequences of this defect are seen in Figure 5–2 and Figure 5–3.

Type IIa hyperlipoproteinemia also may be secondary to myeloma, nephrosis, myxedema, liver disease or excessive dietary intake of cholesterol. Serum cholesterol levels are greater than 300 mg/dl; triglycerides remain normal.

The diet for patients with type IIa hyperlipoproteinemia is difficult to follow, since so many prepared foods contain egg yolk. The diet must be low in cholesterol (less than 300 mg/day), with a high polyunsaturated to saturated fat ratio (P/S) (ideally 1.8–2.8). Fat intake should be restricted to oils or margarines made from safflower, corn, cottonseed or soybean. Safflower or corn oil is preferable, since these oils contain at least 50% linoleic acid. Cholesterol restriction to less than 300 mg/day requires the elimination of egg yolk, organ meats, shrimp, dairy products containing fat and baked goods. To limit saturated fat intake, meat consumption must be restricted to 9 oz cooked meat per

TABLE 5–4.—SAMPLE MENU FOR PATIENTS WITH TYPE IIa HYPERLIPOPROTEINEMIA ON LOW CHOLESTEROL DIET WITH P/S 2.0:1.0 AND 1,800 KCAL

MEAL	WEIGHT (GM)	VITAMIN E (MG)
Breakfast		
½ cup orange juice	100	0.040
¾ cup cornflakes	18	0.020
1 slice toast	20	0.002
1 cup skim milk	246	0.009
1 cup coffee or tea (no cream)		
Lunch or supper		
3 oz chicken (very lean, no skin, prepared	90	0.234
without oil or fat)		
½ cup noodles	80	0.010
½ cup spinach	90	2.250
½ cup lettuce with vinegar	60	0.300
1 slice bread	20	0.002
½ cup unsweetened applesauce	100	0.250
Soft tub margarine		
1 tsp on bread	5	0.580
3 tsp on vegetables or noodles	15	1.740
3 tsp safflower oil (for lettuce)	14	4.872
Coffee or tea (no cream)		
Dinner		
4 oz roast beef (very lean)	120	0.300
1 baked potato	100	0.035
½ cup green beans	62	0.019
½ cup lettuce and tomato with vinegar	60	0.300
1 slice bread	20	0.002
½ cup unsweetened peaches	100	0.250
Soft tub margarine		
1 tsp on bread	5	0.580
3 tsp on vegetables	15	1.740
2 tsp safflower oil (for lettuce and tomato)	9	3.132
Coffee or tea (no cream)		
Bedtime		
1 cup skim milk	246	0.009
1 graham cracker	7	0.023
Total mg Vitamin E		17.279

day. A high P/S can be maintained by consuming three teaspoonsful of corn or safflower oil for every 3 oz cooked meat. Beef, lamb, ham and pork should be limited to 3 oz, three times per week. Carbohydrates are not limited except for calorie control. A sample menu is shown in Table 5-4.

In nonfamilial type IIa hyperlipoproteinemia, diet alone may bring cholesterol within the normal range. With familial type IIa hyperlipoproteinemia, diet alone usually fails, so it should be combined with drug therapy. A 25% reduction in β-lipoprotein and cholesterol may be anticipated by significantly reducing cholesterol intake and substituting polyunsaturated fats. Serum lipids should be determined after 6-8 weeks of dietary therapy.

Type IIb Hyperlipoproteinemia

Type IIb hyperlipoproteinemia shows an increase in β-lipoproteins or LDL and an increase in pre-β-lipoproteins or VLDL. Again, cholesterol levels are greater than 300 mg/dl, and triglycerides are modestly elevated. Frequently, the cholesterol to triglyceride ratio is about 1:1. The diet for patients with this type of hyperlipoproteinemia is low in cholesterol (less than 300 mg/day), with a modified fat ratio (P/S 1.8:2.8) and controlled carbohydrates. Emphasis is on weight reduction to "ideal" weight and maintenance. The rationale for this diet is the same as that for type IIa hyperlipoproteinemia, with the addition of restricting excessive carbohydrate kcal to reduce triglyceride elevation. Concentrated sweets should be eliminated, while fruits, bread, cereal and skim milk are allowed according to the calorie level.

Type III Hyperlipoproteinemia

In type III hyperlipoproteinemia, there is an abnormal form of β-lipoprotein. Both cholesterol and triglycerides are elevated, with concentrations of 350-800 mg/dl. Dietary treatment consists of controlled carbohydrate (40% kcal), controlled and modified fat (40% kcal, with P/S 1:1), less than 300 mg cholesterol per day and reduction of kcal until the patient achieves "ideal" weight. Kilocalories for maintenance of "ideal" weight are then determined. If the overweight patient reduces, endogenous VLDL production will decrease. To achieve the dietary restriction, 2 to 3 oz servings of *lean* meat per day is recommended; the number of servings of fat vary with the kcal level. Animal fats and shortenings are not allowed; only vegetable oils and margarines made from them are allowed. Egg yolks, organ meats and shrimp must be eliminated to restrict cholesterol intake. To control the carbohydrate portion of the diet, concentrated sweets are eliminated, and fruits are restricted to three servings per day. Bread, cereals and skim milk are allowed according to kcal level.

Type IV Hyperlipoproteinemia

CASE PRESENTATION. — M. G. is a 49-year-old woman who was first seen in June, 1972, with the chief complaint of substernal pain. Evaluation revealed an acute anteroseptal myocardial infarction.

Past medical history was negative for hypertension. The patient had a hysterectomy at age 28 and had received "hormones" occasionally since that time.

Family history was negative for heart disease, other degenerative vascular disease and diabetes mellitus.

On physical examination, the patient weighed 60 kg and was 156 cm tall. Pulse was 72 beats/min and regular, and blood pressure was 90/60 mm Hg. The patient was in mild heart failure.

Laboratory work revealed enzymes and electrocardiographic changes compatible with myocardial infarction. The 2-hour postprandial blood sugar was 102 mg/dl. The patient had type IV hyperlipoproteinemia, with 211 mg/dl cholesterol and 185 mg/dl triglycerides. A glucose tolerance test was not done because of the recent infarction. Serum true thyroxin was normal.

The patient was instructed in a type IV hyperlipoproteinemic diet. When she was seen in June 1973, her weight was 50 kg. Her lipoprotein electrophoresis pattern had returned to normal, and serum triglycerides were 80 mg/dl.

Type IV hyperlipoproteinemia is associated with premature atherosclerosis, as was seen in this patient. It is the most common type of hyperlipoproteinemia.

Type IV hyperlipoproteinemia shows an increase in pre-β-lipoprotein or VLDL. Cholesterol levels may be normal, but triglycerides are elevated. The diet for patients with this type of hyperlipoproteinemia is controlled in carbohydrate (40% of kcal), modified in fat and moderately restricted in cholesterol (300–500 mg/day). Again, emphasis is on weight reduction to "ideal" weight and maintenance. Restricting the use of excessive carbohydrate kcal reduces triglyceride elevation. Fats are not limited in this diet but are changed to polyunsaturates to achieve P/S 1:1 as in the diet for patients with type III hyperlipoproteinemia. Dairy products containing fat should be avoided, and meats should be lean. Egg yolks should be limited to three per week and cheese to 2 oz per week. Restriction of alcohol intake also has been advised as a means of reducing triglyceride elevation.

Type IV hyperlipoproteinemia is most common in patients with impaired carbohydrate tolerance. Many studies have shown that sucrose may induce increased formation of pre-β-lipoprotein. This abnormality also can be seen in diabetic patients with insulinopenia due to increased mobilization of fatty acids, which are the substrate for triglyceride formation.

Type V Hyperlipoproteinemia

CASE PRESENTATION.—P. L. is a 54-year-old white female who has had 18 hospitalizations for attacks of abdominal pain reported to be pancreatitis. Marked hyperlipidemia was noted at the time of these attacks.

Thirteen years ago, diabetes was discovered, when the patient was evaluated for fatigue. Even though she was gaining weight at the time, she was started on insulin. Currently, she takes 25 units lente insulin in the A.M. and 10 u/ml in the P.M.

Physical examination revealed an obese woman in no acute distress, with weight 84.6 kg, height 157 cm, pulse 80 beats/min, and blood pressure 160/80 mm Hg. No other positive physical findings were found.

Laboratory results revealed CBC, UA, electrolytes, BUN, creatinine, thyroxin and liver function normal. Fasting blood sugar was 188 mg/dl; serum cholesterol was 256 mg/dl; and triglycerides 1,032 mg/dl. The lipoprotein electrophoresis pattern was described as type V.

The patient was discharged on an 800 kcal, 74 gm carbohydrate, 60 gm protein, 31 gm fat diet.

Three years later, the patient's weight was 77 kg. There has been modest improvement in serum lipids, with 202 mg/dl cholesterol and 704 mg/dl triglycerides.

In type V hyperlipoproteinemia, there is an increase in chylomicrons and pre-β-lipoproteins. Plasma triglycerides are elevated, from 1,000 to 6,000 mg/dl; cholesterol is elevated to a lesser degree. Dietary treatment consists of restricted and modified fat (30% kcal), controlled carbohydrate (50% kcal) and moderately restricted cholesterol (300–500 mg/day). Emphasis is on weight reduction until the patient achieves "ideal" weight. The rationale for this diet is the same as that for type IV hyperlipoproteinemia, with the additional consideration that the patient with type V hyperlipoproteinemia who eats too much fat may have an increase in plasma triglycerides. Meat should be lean; fat should be limited in amount and exclude animal fats, hydrogenated shortenings and coconut oil; egg yolks should be limited to three per week; dairy products containing fat should be avoided. Fruit should be restricted to no more than three servings per day, and concentrated sweets should be avoided. Bread, cereal and skim milk are allowed according to kcal level.

OTHER DIETARY CONSIDERATIONS.—Various food products are used to control dietary lipids. Poultry, game and fish are low in fat, especially if the skins have been removed before cooking. Fish oil is high in polyunsaturated fatty acids. The white of the egg is all protein and contains no cholesterol, while the yolk does contain cholesterol. Oils of fruits, seeds and grains are low in saturated and high in poly-unsaturated fatty acids. Oils containing at least 50% linoleic acid, in order from best to least effective, are safflower, corn, cottonseed and soybean. Hydrogenated oils and margarines are higher in saturated fatty acids, while liquid oils or margarines are higher in polyunsaturated fatty acids. Dietitians counsel patients requiring these foods and make suggestions on specific brands if patients have difficulty distinguishing the difference. There are various low fat, low cholesterol products available on the market today as well as several cookbooks to assist patients in dietary control of hyperlipoproteinemias.

The Vitamin E Question

Tocopherols are widely distributed in foods in an unesterified form and occur in highest concentration in cereal grain oils. Over half the daily intake of α-tocopherol comes from the consumption of various oils and fats of vegetable origin. A deficiency from dietary lack is rare.

Cottonseed, safflower seed and wheat-germ oils are good sources of α-tocopherol (35–163 mg/100 ml). Germ-enriched bread contains about 70 times as much α-tocopherol as white bread. With the exception of oats, processed breakfast cereals retain only 5–15% of their vitamin E content. Meat and poultry are moderately good sources of α-tocopherol (0.3–0.6 mg/100 gm). Eggs and liver are considerably higher (1.1–1.4 mg/100 gm). Butter and cheeses are good sources, while skim milk and nonfat-dry, reconstituted milk are very low. In fruits, α-tocopherol is concentrated in the skin. The tissues of dark-green vegetables are high in α-tocopherol. Refined corn oil (18.7 mg α-tocopherol/100 gm) contains less than half as much α-tocopherol as the lipid from freshly extracted seed corn (41.9 mg/100 gm). Such a difference does not occur in safflower oil.[2]

The estimated average intake of α-tocopherol per capita in the United States is about 14 mg/day, 50% of which is contributed by fats and oils. The 1973 Recommended Dietary Allowances (RDA) state the vitamin E requirement as 15 international units (IU) for the adult male and 12 IU for the adult female. The total vitamin E activity is estimated to be 80% α-tocopherol and 20% other tocopherols. One IU vitamin E is defined as the activity of 1 mg dl-α-tocopherol acetate (1 asymmetric carbon atom in the 2 position). The activity of naturally occurring α-tocopherol, d-α-tocopherol, is 1.49 IU/mg and of its acetate, 1.36 IU/mg. Allowances are based primarily on d-α-tocopherol content of diets.

Patients with a-β-lipoproteinemia are known to have depressed serum levels of tocopherol. With this disease, absorption, transport and perhaps metabolism of lipids and fat-soluble vitamins may be abnormal.[29] If we look at a hypothetical diet for a type IIa hyperlipoproteinemia and check the vitamin E content, we may then compare the vitamin E content to the RDA (see Table 5–4). It is obvious that the diet exceeds the recommended daily requirement for vitamin E. Therefore, supplementation of this vitamin should not be necessary.

Studies Offering Support for Dietary Management

As one might expect, the most fruitful time to alter dietary habits to reduce atherosclerosis is early childhood. Studies of neonates with type II hyperlipoproteinemia demonstrated a mean increase in serum cholesterol from 114 mg/dl at birth to 224 mg/dl at 6 months, when infants were on diets containing normal cholesterol levels.[14] In another seven infants with familial type II hyperlipoproteinemia, a cholesterol-poor, polyunsaturated-rich formula reduced serum cholesterol from 155 mg/dl at birth to 130 mg/dl at 6 months. McGandy and his associates found that when modified fat and cholesterol diets were fed to adolescent boys in a boarding school, their blood cholesterol levels were quickly and appreciably lowered.[28]

There is evidence that dietary management may be beneficial for adults also. Bierenbaum and his co-workers found that over a five-year period 100 men with documented coronary artery disease benefited from a diet containing 28% fat, with saturated fat content below 9% of the total calories and cholesterol intake less than 400 mg per day.[7] This diet resulted in a significant reduction in serum cholesterol and triglyceride levels and a reduction in reinfarction rates. Evans and his associates have also demonstrated a fall in serum cholesterol and triglyceride levels when saturated fat and cholesterol in the diet were substituted by highly unsaturated fatty acids.[11]

Friedman studied patients with elevations of the pre-β-lipoprotein levels and showed a decrease in pre- and postprandial hypertriglyceridemia when the intake of simple sugar was reduced.[12]

In some individuals, fructose intake may affect triglyceride formation. MacDonald has shown that fructose consumption may lead to inordinately high serum fructose levels in some people, resulting in increased triglyceride levels.[22]

An important question remains unanswered: Will altering the diet increase longevity for patients who already have arterial disease? Direct information on man is difficult to obtain, since we are all very hesitant to use invasive procedures to do follow-up studies.

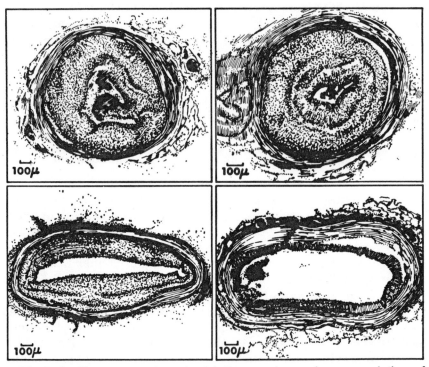

Fig 5-4.—Top, encroachment of intima on lumen by accumulation of lipid-laden macrophages and fibrosis proliferation and cellular breakdown in coronary arteries from monkeys on a diet high in saturated fats. **Bottom,** regression of atherosclerosis after several weeks on a diet low in cholesterol and with P/S ratio of 2:1. (From Armstrong, M. L., Warner, E. D., and Connor, W. E.: Circ. Res. 27:59, 1970. Used by permission of the American Heart Association, Inc.)

Armstrong and his coworkers have convincing evidence that feeding a low cholesterol, high polyunsaturated fat diet to monkeys with established atherosclerosis causes regression of the atheromatous plaques (Fig 5-4).[3] Jagannathan has shown a definite exchange of cholesterol between plasma and severely atherosclerotic human arteries, which suggests the possibility that cholesterol can be mobilized and that regression of atheromatous lesions in man is possible.[18] This gives encouragement to the individual with known coronary artery disease.

In reality, there is as much evidence to support the usefulness of dietary management of coronary artery disease as there is to support that of coronary bypass procedures. Reason would tend to make us suspect that dietary management should be beneficial. The practical problem is that most people are unwilling to alter their eating habits until catastrophy has struck and the disease is far advanced.

Controversial Studies and Articles

In contrast to the studies reviewed previously, Moutafis and Myant found that a patient's plasma cholesterol concentration remained essentially unchanged on a high cholesterol intake even though the diagnosis of type II hyperlipoproteinemia was established.[30]

Other dietary considerations related to hyperlipoproteinemia have been suggested by some investigators. Spittle found that cholesterol levels tended to fall in *healthy* people when vitamin D was added to a normal diet. In patients with a history of atherosclerosis, serum cholesterol increased when vitamin C supplements were given.[36] Malhotra suggested certain dietary changes which would produce a greater amount of short-chain fatty acids and a decrease in the density and complexity of chylomicrons. The recommendations were as follows: (1) increase the amount of cellulose; (2) increase the consumption of fermented milk products; (3) masticate foods properly; and (4) cook by methods that reduce the size of fat globules (as frying with turmeric powder).[24]

The mechanism of alcohol-induced hypertriglyceridemia is not well understood. However, in a study reported by Fry and others on a 44-year-old white male who had had a myocardial infarction, feeding 25% kcal as alcohol produced a rapid increase in serum triglycerides from fasting levels of 547 mg/dl to 750–900 mg/dl. The diet formula contained 40% carbohydrate and 20% fat. The lipoprotein electrophoresis showed an accentuation of the pre-β band. When dietary carbohydrate was increased to 65% total kcal, there was a threefold increase in triglyceride concentration from 288 to 898 mg/dl on the 10th day.[13]

Dietary management of the hyperlipoproteinemias still remains controversial, since there are few, if any, follow-up studies to confirm beneficial effects. Patients should be followed, their serum lipids should be checked frequently and assessment of dietary treatment should be made. No one likes to follow a diet needlessly or without results. If the diet proves successful, the patient should receive reinforcement and encouragement to continue following a specific dietary regimen.

REFERENCES
1. Abel, E. J., and Powell, R. C.: An approach to the dietary management of hyperlipemia, J. Indiana State Med. Assoc. 64:827, 1971.

2. Ames, S. R.: Tocopherols: Occurrence in foods, in Sebrell, W. H., and Harris, R. S. (eds.): *The Vitamins* (New York: Academic Press, 1972).

3. Armstrong, M. L., Warner, E. D., and Conner, W. E.: Regression of coronary atheromatosis in Rhesus monkeys, Circ. Res. 27:59, 1970.

4. Bagdade, J. D., and Bierman, E. L.: Diagnosis and dietary treatment of blood lipid disorders, Med. Clin. North Am. 54:1383, 1970.

5. Bateson, M. C., and Lant, A. F.: Dietary potassium and diuretic therapy, Lancet 2:381, 1973.

6. Beaumont, J. L., et al.: Classification of hyperlipidemias and hyperlipoproteinemias, Bull. W.H.O. 43:891, 1970.

7. Bierenbaum, M. L., et al.: The 5-year experience of modified fat diets on younger men with coronary heart disease, Circulation 43:943, 1970.

8. Bolinger, R., et al.: Metabolic balance of obese subjects during fasting, Arch. Intern. Med. 118:3, 1966.

9. Brown, H. B.: Specifying food products for fat control, Hospitals 46:126, 1972.

10. Dahl, L. K.: Salt and hypertension, Am. J. Clin. Nutr. 25:231, 1972.

11. Evans, D. W., Turner, S. M., and Ghosh, P.: Feasibility of long-term plasma cholesterol reduction by diet, Lancet 1:172, 1972.

12. Friedman, M., et al.: Effect of low sugar intake upon blood lipids and insulin levels of hyperlipemic subjects, Proc. Soc. Exp. Biol. Med. 135:785, 1970.

13. Fry, M. M., et al.: Intensification of hypertriglyceridemia by either alcohol or carbohydrate, Am. J. Clin. Nutr. 26:798, 1973.

14. Glueck, C. J., and Tsang, R. C.: Pediatric familial type II hyperlipoproteinemia: Effects of diet on plasma cholesterol in the first year of life, Am. J. Clin. Nutr. 25:224, 1972.

15. Goldstein, J. L., and Brown, M. S.: Hyperlipidemia in coronary heart disease: A biochemical genetic approach, J. Lab. Clin. Med. 85:15, 1975.

16. Goodhart, R. S., and Shils, M. E.: *Modern Nutrition in Health and Disease, Dietotherapy* (5th ed.; Philadelphia: Lea & Febiger, 1973), p. 888.

17. Grande, F., Anderson, J. T., and Keys, A.: Diets of different fatty acid composition producing identical serum cholesterol levels in man, Am. J. Clin. Nutr. 25:53, 1972.

18. Jagannathan, S. N., et al.: The turnover of cholesterol in human atherosclerotic arteries, J. Clin. Invest. 54:366, 1975.

19. Leren, P.: The Oslo diet-heart study: Eleven-year report, Circulation 42:935, 1970.

20. Levy, R. I., et al.: Dietary and drug treatment of primary hyperlipoproteinemia, Ann. Intern. Med. 77:267, 1972.

21. Lewis, B.: Diet and plasma lipoproteins, Clin. Sci. 40:16P, 1971.

22. MacDonald, I., and Turner, L. J.: Serum glucose and fructose levels after sucrose meals in atherosclerosis, Nutr. Metab. 13:168, 1971.

23. Maha, G. E.: Diet and drug therapy for hyperlipoproteinemia, Med. Times 99:49, 1971.

24. Malhotra, S. L.: Dietary factors and ischemic heart disease, Am. J. Clin. Nutr. 24:1195, 1971.

25. Mayer, J.: Low sodium diets, I. Mild restriction, Postgrad. Med. 49:193, 1971.

26. Mayer, J.: Low sodium diets, II. Severe restriction, Postgrad. Med. 50:49, 1971.
27. McAllister, R. G.: Chronic salt excess and hypertension: A cultural epidemic, J. Tenn. Med. Assoc. 64:581, 1971.
28. McGandy, R. B., et al.: Dietary regulation of blood cholesterol in adolescent males: A pilot study, Am. J. Clin. Nutr. 25:61, 1972.
29. Melborn, D. K.: Vitamin E: Who needs it? R.I. Med. J. 57:100, 1974.
30. Moutafis, C. D., and Myant, N. B.: The effect of prolonged high cholesterol intake on cholesterol metabolism in man with type II hyperlipoproteinemia, Clin. Sci. 40:19P, 1971.
31. Quintao, E., Grundy, S. M., and Ahrens, E. H.: Effects of dietary cholesterol on the regulation of total body cholesterol in man, J. Lipid Res. 12: 233, 1971.
32. Reiser, R.: Saturated fat in the diet and serum cholesterol concentration: A critical examination of the literature, Am. J. Clin. Nutr. 26:524, 1973.
33. Saunders, E.: Dietary salt (sodium chloride) intake and arterial hypertension. Part 2, Md. State Med. J. 19:109, 1970.
34. Schattenberg, T. T., and Brandenburg, R. O.: Nutrition and cardiovascular disease, Med. Clin. North Am. 54:1449, 1970.
35. Schonfeld, G., and Kudzma, D. J.: Type IV hyperlipoproteinemia: A critical appraisal, Arch. Intern. Med. 132:55, 1973.
36. Spittle, C. R.: Atherosclerosis and vitamin D, Lancet 1:1280, 1971.
37. Swaye, P. S., Gifford, R. W., and Berrettoni, J. N.: Dietary salt and essential hypertension, Am. J. Cardiol. 29:33, 1972.
38. Tobian, L.: Some aspects of the relationship of salt and hypertension, Trans. Am. Clin. Climatol. Assoc. 78:153, 1966.
39. Walter, A. R.: Sugar intake and coronary heart disease, Atherosclerosis 14: 137, 1971.
40. Witting, L. A.: The role of polyunsaturated fatty acids in determining vitamin E requirement, Ann. N.Y. Acad. Sci. 203:192, 1972.
41. Youngstrom, K. A.: Low sodium diet: A personal experience of its benefits and pleasures, J. Kans. Med. Soc. 82:263, 1971.

Chapter 6 / Diet and Nutrition for the Surgical Patient

FOR THE MAJORITY of individuals who are subjected to a single, uncomplicated, major surgical procedure, immediate preoperative and postoperative nutrition is simply a program of parenteral infusion. This intravenous "nutrition" is designed to maintain the blood circulating volume and to provide water, glucose, salt and potassium to prevent dehydration and electrolyte imbalance. In the well-nourished and otherwise healthy patient, glucose in the infusion prevents protein breakdown, beyond that which usually results from the stress or trauma of surgery. Generally, body reserves of protein and fat can sustain most patients for a week or more of inadequate caloric and protein intake without grave consequences.

For a significant minority of surgical patients, a nutrition program must be planned carefully preoperatively, as well as postoperatively. Patients who are severely debilitated and malnourished as a result of chronic disease and those who have been unwilling or unable to eat adequately for a prolonged period of time due to trauma, sepsis or other complications have marked weight loss and severe reduction in skeletal mass and total body protein. Such patients are poor operative risks and require serious attention to nutritional management in the preoperative period. Because it had not been determined whether malnutrition causes formation of a poor scar or slow rate of normal healing, Temple and his co-workers studied malnutrition produced by the short gut syndrome in rats. Their results were as follows: (1) improved nutrition led to greater survival of animals, but ultimate wound healing was indistinguishable from that of normal controls; (2) early weakness resulted from slow healing rather than poor scar formation; and (3) nutrition played an important role in early strength and survival but not in ultimate wound healing.[28]

Preoperative Nutrition

A state of good nutrition before surgery is important and should be determined by physical examination, laboratory data and dietary history. If the patient is in a poor nutritional state, surgery may have to be postponed while measures are instituted to improve nutrition. Calories are important, but even more important is protein. If a patient is unable to eat food, then oral hyperalimentation with high protein supplements or high nitrogen elemental diets should be tried. If oral hyperalimentation does not provide the solution, then it may be necessary to use the parenteral or intravenous route. Total parenteral nutrition (TPN) and elemental diets will be discussed at length later in this chapter. The objective of preoperative nutrition is to achieve good body weight and adequate muscle mass and obtain normal serum albumin and total protein levels before stress induces protein breakdown and nitrogen loss.

At the opposite end of the spectrum is the obese patient. If time permits, surgery may have to be postponed while measures are instituted to reduce the patient's weight. The obese patient is an obvious surgical risk, as is the undernourished patient. Excessive fat accumulation makes surgery difficult and wound healing slow. A diet restricted in calories but adequate in protein, vitamins and minerals should be the preoperative program for these patients.

Immediate preoperative nutrition for all patients requires clearing the gastrointestinal tract of partially digested food to prevent vomiting and possible aspiration of food into the bronchi during postoperative recovery. Therefore, depending on the nature of the surgery, clear liquids are taken for a specified period of time. Then, nothing by mouth is the usual order from midnight preceding surgery. Gatorade and Citrotein, both low residue liquids, have been used up to three hours prior to surgery without any side effects. These liquids help relieve thirst, supply a few calories and add small amounts of electrolytes. Citrotein also supplies some amino acids.

Postoperative Nutrition

Until peristalsis returns, food and fluids cannot be given by mouth. However, fluid and electrolyte replacements must be made to prevent dehydration and shock. In addition, a minimum number of calories can be provided through glucose. These replacements are made by intravenous feedings. When orders are written for parenteral fluid and electrolyte therapy, baseline requirements, abnormal losses and deficits or excesses should be taken into consideration.

Normal baseline parenteral water requirements vary from 1,500 to 3,000 ml/day, depending on age, sex and body cell mass. Factors such as fever, sweating and increased metabolism increase insensible water loss and thereby increase the water requirement in parenteral feeding.[27] Normal sodium intake in the adult is 100 mEq/day or higher, but sodium is retained after surgery due to increased tubular reabsorption produced by aldosterone. From 5 to 7 days after surgery, sodium diuresis occurs. Therefore, the accepted clinical practice is to provide about 80 mEq of sodium in the first 24 hours postoperatively. Sodium is supplied in 500 ml of normal saline and about 1.5 L of water as dextrose solution.[31] Normal potassium intake is about 80 mEq/day, but potassium excretion is increased in the urine for the first 2–3 days after surgery. An allowance of 40 mEq/L excreted urine is recommended before potassium is added in the form of potassium chloride.[31] Generally, body stores of calcium are adequate, and it is rare to consider the need for giving calcium to postoperative patients in any way other than in food when they begin to eat. Magnesium is not given intravenously except to patients with liver disease or intestinal malabsorption or those on prolonged intravenous infusions.[31]

The administration of carbohydrate as dextrose or glucose will not prevent complete breakdown of body cell mass, even when 200 to 400 gm/day are provided. However, 100 to 125 gm of glucose/day parenterally will prevent nearly half the nitrogen loss resulting from catabolism of lean body mass.[27] In addition, B-complex vitamins and vitamin C should be administered parenterally, especially to patients who are not well nourished due to prolonged sepsis or small bowel disease.[31]

Abnormal losses of water, electrolytes and plasma proteins, both externally and internally, must be considered also in evaluating fluid and electrolyte determinations. Losses from the gastrointestinal tract include water and electrolytes and various amounts of protein through diarrhea. Internal fluid shifts occur with burns, crush injuries, peritonitis, soft tissue damage and wound infection. If the volume of sequestered fluid is significantly large, it must be replaced just as an external loss. However, sequestered fluid eventually will return to the circulation, posing the potential problem of fluid and electrolyte overload.[27]

The third consideration in fluid and electrolyte therapy is the replacement of deficits of water and electrolytes to restore function after major losses and the recognition and treatment of excessive fluid volumes or concentrations of electrolytes. Problems that must be considered and treated are acute or chronic dehydration, desiccation, chronic overexpansion of extracellular fluid, hypertonicity due to solute loading or overhydration, hypotonicity and water intoxication.[27]

Patients who are well nourished and reasonably healthy prior to surgery and who have a single or relatively uncomplicated major surgical procedure require very little modification in nutritional care following surgery. Oral feedings are initiated as soon as possible after bowel sounds have returned. Clear liquids are offered at first; then, the patient may progress to his normal diet as tolerated. It is not un-common for a patient to be on a general diet by the 2d or 3d postopera-tive day.

Certain groups of surgical patients require a carefully planned pro-gram of postoperative nutrition. In addition, their intakes should be diligently monitored and assessed. These groups are: first, cardiac surgical patients; second, gastrointestinal surgical patients. Metabolic changes after open heart surgery follow the same pattern as the usual injury. Therefore, nutritional status and metabolic balance during the postoperative period should be a significant factor in the patient's re-covery. Manners conducted a study in a clinical setting to assess the nutritional balance of 12 adult patients during seven days following open heart surgery. Intravenous or oral fluids were prescribed on the day of operation and on the first postoperative day. After the first post-operative day, intake was not limited; patients were allowed unre-stricted food and water by mouth. Nine patients had low food intake and negative nitrogen balance during the 7 days following open heart surgery. Average values indicated that a 65 kg man excreted 104 ml more urine per day than the amount of water taken in, consumed 800 kcal per day, with a nitrogen intake of 4.7 gm/day, and had a urinary nitrogen loss of 10.7 gm/day. Average calorie intake of 12.1 kcal/kg/day was by no means optimal.[19]

It is unlikely that a cardiac surgical patient will meet his total ener-gy requirement, let alone his nitrogen requirement, if he is placed on a diet "ad lib." As indicated in Manners' study, two patients with a caloric intake of 10.1 kcal/kg/day and 8.4 kcal/kg/day remained in the hospital 41 days and 58 days, respectively. Both had wound infection and large negative nitrogen balance.[19] No doubt, the poor nutritional status of these patients contributed to their prolonged hospitalization. Progress to mobilization and graded exercise was retarded, and recov-ery of the cardiovascular system was delayed. Therefore, it seems evi-dent that nutritional support of cardiac surgical patients is imperative. Oral feeding is established within 1 to 2 days after surgery so that supplemental feedings to the usual hospital meals can easily achieve a better nutritional status.

Abel and his co-workers evaluated 44 malnourished cardiac surgical patients. Twenty-four were considered controls, and 20 received immediate postoperative parenteral hyperalimentation. Five days of nutritional therapy had no notable effect on morbidity and mortality rates. The investigators concluded that postoperative repletion of nu-trients did not effectively reverse development of complications, even though preoperative malnutrition was associated with a poorer result after cardiac surgery.[2]

Following surgery of the mouth, throat or neck, alterations in the type or method of feeding may have to be made. Liquid or semiliquid feedings are usually required. McKeown discussed the nutritional state of the patient who has been treated with surgery for esophageal carcinoma. Emphasis was placed on a diet high in protein, calories, vitamin C and the B-complex vitamins for the healing of parietal and visceral structures and the prevention of stomal leak after esophagectomy. If oral feeding is impossible, intravenous therapy (hyperalimentation) is necessary. Gastrostomy or jejunostomy may be advocated for some patients; but it is better to avoid this form of feeding, since it interferes with subsequent surgical procedures and adds to the risk of infection.[21] Ross discussed the importance of some of the same points in the nutritional management of patients receiving radiotherapy for carcinoma of the esophagus. He stressed the importance of improving and maintaining the patient's nutritional state from the outset of treatment.[25]

Following gastric surgery, the dietary regimen commonly includes small, frequent feedings and excludes highly seasoned or spicy foods, coffee and alcohol. Due to the need for very small feedings and frequent discomfort following meals, patients are often unable to consume an adequate amount of nutrients. Nutritional supplements to fortify inadequate intake may be indicated. Bradley and his associates reported on the ability of ten patients to ingest and absorb adequate amounts of nutrients following total gastrectomy and the results of metabolic balance studies. In the hospital setting, the amount of food ingested was greater than the amount required for maintenance of ideal body weight. Weight gain and positive nitrogen balance occurred, even though there was mild malabsorption of fat and nitrogen. When patients returned to the home environment, food intake decreased significantly. Bradley concluded that the most common mechanism responsible for postoperative malnutrition was inadequate intake rather than malabsorption.[4]

Following surgery of the small or large intestine, solid foods may not be tolerated for various periods of time. Motor activity of the colon in the immediate postoperative period was studied in 36 patients: 6 after partial gastrectomy, 1 after total gastrectomy, 6 after vagotomy and pyloroplasty, 1 after cholecystojejunostomy, 2 after left hemicolectomy, 6 after cholecystectomy, 2 after exploratory laparotomy, 4 after retropubic prostatectomy, 1 after herniorrhaphy, 2 after mastectomy, 1 after thyroidectomy, 2 after ligation of varicose veins and 1 after transurethral resection of the prostate. Colonic activity did not return until 40–48 hours after abdominal surgery but returned within 16 hours following surgery that was not performed on the abdomen. Length of surgery and amount of postoperative analgesia had no significant effect on duration of colonic ileus. Gaseous distention after laparotomy was confined to the colon.[33] This study indicates the variation from case to case on the return of bowel sounds. Obviously, gastrointestinal surgical patients must go without oral feeding for a longer period of time.

Clear liquid diets are often used in combination with parenteral feedings. In addition, a chemically defined, low residue diet may be initiated. These diets will be discussed in detail later in this chapter. They have the advantage of providing adequate intake of essential nutrients in a readily absorbable form, while reducing stool volume to a minimum. With time, the diet can generally be advanced to include the patient's regular food tolerances. Severe malabsorption problems resulting from surgical procedures must be handled on an individual basis to develop a diet that responds to special needs.

Mason and Printen reported their work with nine female patients who had previously undergone end-to-side anastomosis in intestinal bypass surgery (14 in. jejunum to 4 in. ileum). Patients were readmitted 5 to 48 months postoperatively with diarrhea, nausea, vomiting and profound weakness. They had lost from 65 to 151 lb, and physical and laboratory findings were compatible with active liver disease. All but one patient retained fluid, some massively, and had ascites and peripheral edema. Five patients were so severely depleted of body protein and so edematous that prolonged TPN was necessary. As nutrition improved, personality changes were noted. The patients became alert, interested, cooperative and active participants. Thus, profound malnutrition of patients after bypass surgery requires close observation and treatment.[20]

Chemically Defined or "Elemental" Diets

The development of chemically defined oral or enteral diets evolved from the use of chemically defined intravenous nutrition. Though the first diets were developed in the late 1960s, it was not until the early 1970s that clinical investigations and their results were reported in the literature. Thus, the use of these chemically formulated, bulk-free diets is relatively new. Commercial diets are improperly labeled "elemental," because most are not composed of the "elements." A chemically defined diet (CDD) is a nutritionally complete predigested liquid diet that is precisely formulated to support growth, development and tissue repletion in normal and debilitated patients.[16, 27, 29, 35]

Nutrients provided by CDD require little or no digestion, are readily and almost completely absorbed in the upper small intestine (relatively small portion of the gut) and provide minimum residue to the large bowel. A study of the use of Vivonex-100 on dogs showed that nutritional status could be maintained or improved without major stimulation of the pancreas, insofar as pancreatic enzyme response was concerned.[22]

Chemically defined diets have been shown to be of special benefit and are indicated for use in preoperative bowel preparation; postoperative management of colonic and rectal surgery; management of gastrointestinal fistulas, inflammatory bowel disease, malabsorption and short gut syndromes and pancreatitis; protein-calorie malnutrition and accelerated catabolic state; and vascular diseases, trauma and neoplasms of the gastrointestinal tract. Their use in offering greater nutritional support to cachectic and burned patients is increasing markedly.[18, 27, 29, 30, 35]

When a portion of functional intestine is available for absorption, utilization of CDD avoids the risks of total parenteral nutrition and provides all essential nutrients. By virtue of enteral administration, CDD offers these advantages: (1) avoidance of infection; (2) reduced "pain" in preparation, i.e., sterile technique is not as important; (3) addition of fats to supply essential fatty acids; and (4) greater leeway in provision of micronutrients.[29]

Methods of administration of CDD are oral and intragastric tube feeding. Due to their chemical nature, most CDDs are not palatable and are not well tolerated by patients when taken orally. In addition, it becomes more difficult to monitor amounts ingested to avoid high osmolality. If the oral route is chosen, only small amounts (100–150 ml) should be given at a time. Over a 16-hour period, it is possible to provide 2,000 cal with the ingestion of 2,000 ml CDD. In addition, the patient should be receiving 40 gm protein or more.[27]

A technique for continual administration of an elemental diet by catheter was developed and reported by Page and his co-workers. They found this method adequate to maintain good nutritional support for patients who could not manage the diet orally. If a nasogastric feeding was indicated, a 16-gauge, 24-in. polyethylene catheter was used. Alimentation was initiated with 25% weight/volume solution, 1 cal/ml, at a rate of 50 ml/hr. The rate was increased by 25 ml/hr up to a total of 125 ml/hr and 3,000 cal/24 hrs. If a jejunostomy feeding was indicated, a 16-gauge, 36-in. polyethylene catheter was used. Alimentation was initiated with 10% weight/volume solution at 50 ml/hr and increased by 25 ml/hr each day up to daily fluid requirements. Then, the concentration was increased by 5% weight/volume/day until max-

TABLE 6-1.—COMPARISON OF COMPONENTS OF
CHEMICALLY DEFINED DIETS

COMPONENT	VIVONEX	VIVONEX HN	PRECISION LR
Carbohydrate			
gm/1000 kcal	226.0	210.0	224.7
% cal	90.56	82.80	89.89
Type	Glucose Oligosaccharides	Glucose Oligosaccharides	Maltodextrin Sucrose citrate
Lactose	None	None	None
Fat			
gm/1000 kcal	1.4	0.9	0.7
% cal	1.26	0.80	0.63
Type	Safflower oil	Safflower oil	Soy oil Mono- and diglycerides
Essential fatty acids (% total fat)	80	80	
Amino acids	20.4	41.6	23.7
gm/1000 kcal	8.18	16.40	9.48
% cal			
Type	Pure crystalline amino acids	Pure crystalline amino acids	Egg albumin (pasteurized egg white solids)
Osmolality			
mOsm/kg (at standard dilution)	550	800	525 (Orange)
Cost per 1000 kcal	$4.36	$8.38	$2.79

imum tolerance was achieved (generally, 20% weight/volume concentration, 4/5 cal/ml, at 125 ml/hr for 2,400 cal/day). Body weight, intake and output and blood and urine sugars, were monitored daily. Serum electrolytes, BUN and albumin were obtained routinely.[23]

Voitk described intragastric administration somewhat differently and suggested an initial feeding of 1,500 ml, half-strength, given over a 24-hour period. In two days, the same volume of full-strength solution was given. Then, the volume was increased by 500–1,000 ml daily until patient tolerance was reached (usually, 3,000–5,000 ml/24 hours). He suggested either a pump or gravity-controlled drip system for continuous infusion.[29]

There are several possible complications that may arise with use of CDD: (1) aspiration; (2) gastrointestinal disturbances, i.e., nausea and vomiting, cramps and diarrhea and delayed gastric emptying; (3) fluid balance disturbances, i.e., fluid retention, hyperosmolar dehydration and hypertonic nonketotic coma; (4) hyperglycemia; and (5) hypoprothrombinemia. Many of these complications can be avoided if the technique of administration is proper. For nonedematous salt and

TABLE 6–1.—*Continued*

PRECISION MN	PRECISION HN	PRECISION ISOTONIC	FLEXICAL
150.0	206.7	150.0	154.0
59.46	82.84	59.90	60.87
Maltodextrin	Maltodextrin	Glucose	Sucrose
Sucrose citrate	Sucrose citrate	Oligosaccharides	Oligosaccharides
		Sucrose citrate	Sucrose citrate
None	None	None	None
31.0	0.5	31.3	34.0
27.65	0.45	28.12	30.24
Soy oil	Soy oil	Soy oil	Soy oil
Mono- and	Mono- and	Mono- and	MCT oil
diglycerides	diglycerides	diglycerides	Mono- and
			diglycerides
			26.5
32.5	41.7	30.0	22.5
12.89	16.71	11.98	8.89
Egg albumin	Egg albumin	Egg albumin	Hydrolyzed casein
(pasteurized egg	(pasteurized egg	(pasteurized egg	(free amino acids
white solids)	white solids)	white solids)	and small pep-
			tides)
395	557	300	723
			(Flavored)
$3.87	$5.71	$4.76	$3.63

water retention on refeeding cachectic patients, hydrochlorothiazide may be given in doses of 25–50 mg every other day. In addition, the physician must select very carefully the nutrient composition of the diet, keeping in mind the specific needs of each patient. Depending on the underlying disease and any other conditions the patient might have (cardiac, renal or hepatic disease), the concentration and presence of certain nutrients may be deficient or excessive to meet the patient's needs.[18, 27, 29, 35]

There are important differences in the nutritional components of each of the commercially available CDDs. Although carbohydrates contribute the largest percentage of calories, the amount varies widely from brand to brand. The type of carbohydrate also varies from hexose and glucose to complex oligosaccharides. Nitrogen content is derived from pure crystalline amino acids, hydrolyzed casein, egg albumin or "synthetic" amino acids. The optimal form of nitrogen or protein in these diets has not been established. The amount of fat available from these diets differs greatly. Some contain very little, which may lead to essential fatty acid deficiency. Most of the fats in CDDs are derived from safflower, soy or corn oil. However, one brand contains medium-chain triglycerides, which are absorbed directly into the portal system.[18, 27, 29, 35] Table 6–1 shows the composition of the commonly used chemically defined diets and demonstrates the comparisons previously mentioned.

Total Parenteral Nutrition (TPN)

Intravenous feeding was initially developed to give nutritional support after surgery or trauma. However, the basic problem associated with conventional intravenous feeding of 5–10% dextrose in water with electrolytes was the inability to provide sufficient calories to prevent tissue catabolism and protein loss. Therefore, even a well-nourished patient could not be maintained for prolonged periods of time on conventional parenteral feeding. Though the term "hyperalimentation," or total parenteral nutrition, appeared in the literature in the mid- to late-1960s, it was mistakenly interpreted to mean administration of total nutrition by vein. The term, when broken down into its prefix—hyper—and route—alimentation—should refer to the administration of calories in *excess* of those needed for nourishment, support or sustenance. Thus, the phrase "total parenteral nutrition" appears more accurate in reference to providing to a specific patient required calories and nutrients parenterally, rather than orally or by tube-fed routes.

When enteral feeding is impossible, ill-advised or inadequate, long-term TPN can be an effective adjunct in the treatment of many diseases or disorders. Use of TPN is indicated for surgical patients who are

TABLE 6–2.—INDICATIONS FOR TOTAL
PARENTERAL NUTRITION

Malnutrition	Failure to thrive
Malabsorption	Chronic diarrhea
Chronic vomiting	Gastrointestinal obstruction
Ulcer disease	Granulomatous enterocolitis
Ulcerative colitis	Regional enteritis
Pancreatitis	Severe anorexia nervosa
Indolent wounds and	Reversible liver failure
decubitus ulcers	Acute and chronic renal failure
Diverticulitis	Burns
Alimentary track fistula	Complicated trauma or surgery
Alimentary tract anomalies	Protein-losing gastroenteropathy
Hypermetabolic states	Malignant disease
Short bowel syndrome	(adjunctive therapy)
Nonterminal coma	

malnourished or who have complicated surgery, short bowel syndrome or indolent wounds.[3, 9, 10, 11, 12, 13, 27] A list of indications for use of TPN appears in Table 6-2.

Although earlier methods of intravenous feeding using relatively small concentrations of nutrients per volume of involved fluid were administered through peripheral veins, TPN requires infusion into a large diameter, central vein, the superior vena cava via the subclavian vein. The concentrated nutrient solution can be rapidly diluted by high blood flow and thereby sent to the periphery in isotonic concentration, which minimizes the occurrence of phlebitis or thrombosis. The total volume of fluid administered is equal to daily water requirements and is infused at a constant rate over a 24-hour period, which allows maximum utilization of the nutrients and minimum renal excretion.[11, 27] Rutten and his associates studied 13 patients to determine an optimal hyperalimentation infusion rate and found that the delivery of 1.76 basal energy expenditure was necessary to produce positive nitrogen balance with 95% confidence in patients with mild to moderate catabolic states.[26]

In general, the average adult patient should receive 3 L or 3,000 ml of solution per day, which supplies about 3,000 kcal. The basic nutrient solution is approximately 30% solute, 20% of which is dextrose or glucose, 5% amino acids or protein hydrolysates and 5% vitamins and minerals. The formula must be established according to individual patient needs; so there is no "standard" formula.[10, 11, 12] In terms of grams of protein and dextrose and mEq of minerals or electrolytes, the aim is to provide at least 100 gm of protein in the form of amino acids or hydrolysates, 500-650 gm of dextrose or glucose, 125-150 mEq of sodium, 75-125 mEq of potassium, 8-24 mEq of magnesium, 4½-9 mEq of calcium and 45-60 mEq of phosphate.[11] The formula can be prepared in bulk under a laminar flow hood in the hospital pharmacy. Vitamin and iron preparations are given separately, either in 1 unit of solution per day or intravenously or intramuscularly. Vitamins and iron are given once a day in the following amounts: 5 ml multiple vitamin infusion (routine), 5-10 mg vitamin K (optional), 10-30 μg vitamin B_{12} (optional), 0.5-1.5 ml folic acid (optional) and 1.0-3.0 mg iron (dextriferron).[11] The solution for children is quite different, since their needs are different. Table 6-3 shows the comparison of parenteral solutions for adults and children.

Two hydrolyzed proteins and crystalline amino acids are used. Fibrin and casein are complete proteins, which are hydrolyzed to produce amino acids, dipeptides and some tripeptides. This solution is usually dialyzed to prevent any large particles that may cause adverse

TABLE 6–3.—COMPOSITION OF TOTAL
PARENTERAL NUTRITION

	ADULT	CHILD
Composition	165 gm anhydrous dextrose (USP) + 860 ml 5% dextrose in 5% protein hydrolysate	400 ml 5% dextrose in 5% fibrin hydrolysate + 250 ml 50% dextrose
Preparation	Sterilization through 0.22 Å membrane filter under laminar flow, filtered air hood	
Volume	1,000 ml	650 ml
Calories	1,000 kcal	660 kcal
Dextrose	208 gm	145 gm
Hydrolysates	43 gm	20 gm
Nitrogen	6 gm	2.79 gm
Sodium	~ 8 mEq	–
Potassium	~ 14 mEq	–
Additions to each unit of base solution (mEq)		
Sodium	40–50	20
Potassium	30–40	25
Phosphorus	15–20 (optional)	25
Calcium	4–9 (optional)	20
Magnesium	8–12	10
Additions to only one unit daily		
Multiple vitamin infusion	5 ml (routine)	4 ml
Vitamin K	5–10 mg (optional)	–
Vitamin B_{12}	10–30 μg (optional)	1 ml
Folic acid	0.5–1.5 mg (optional)	–
Iron	1.0–3.0 mg (optional)	–
Trace elements	–	1 ml

reactions. Certain side effects, such as fever and urticarial rashes, have been observed with protein hydrolysates. Acidosis is less of a problem with use of hydrolysates. The pH is about 5.5, which is slightly acidic, but this is not a significant titratable acidity. Approximately 10% total nitrogen in hydrolysates is in the form of ammonia nitrogen, but this load can be handled well in patients without liver disease. Crystalline amino acids, on the other hand, tend to cause hyperammonemia, probably due to the lower arginine content. In addition, crystalline amino acids may cause hyperchloremic metabolic acidosis, because 80% or more of the total amino acids in some solutions are in the form of chloride or hydrochloride salts. Though synthetic amino acids are more difficult to use because of various metabolic problems, they decrease the problem of allergies and also supply more usable nitrogen per liter.[11, 12, 34]

Intravenous fat emulsions and their use have been quite controversial. Until recently, a parenteral form of essential fatty acids was not available in the United States because of the lack of an approved intravenous emulsion with polyunsaturated fat. Dudrick stated that the lack of fat in these parenteral solutions has not caused any major or insurmountable problems for his patients, but he admitted a few cases of fatty acid deficiency had been reported in the literature recently.[11] A study reported in the literature in 1975 revealed that, depending on the severity of the operation, use of fat after surgery was increased and return to normal fat use was related to regaining an adequate caloric intake. Therefore, it was concluded that fat is the body's natural source of energy after injury and should be used to provide calories in parenteral feedings.[15] Zohrab and his associates reported that with a balanced parenteral alimentation containing lipid the fistula closed, symptoms of imflammatory gastrointestinal diseases subsided and malnutrition was corrected.[36] Yeo and his co-workers studied fat added to total intravenous nutrition and compared it to glucose total intravenous nutrition. Patients receiving fat did not gain as much weight as those on glucose due to fewer total calories. Fewer calories could be administered because of the Food and Drug Administration's limitation on the amount of fat administered. The 3 gm/kg/day limitation is probably far below the level that can be metabolized. Four of six patients receiving the fat emulsion developed positive nitrogen balance when fed 6–8 gm of nitrogen per sq m/day. However, positive nitrogen balance was also achieved in four patients on glucose total intravenous nutrition.[34] In this study, fat and glucose appeared to be equally good sources of calories in total intravenous nutrition.

Intravenous fat solutions have advantages over hypertonic glucose solutions, such as more calories per gram, a supply of essential fatty acids and decreased risk of metabolic acidosis. The soybean oil emulsion has minimal side effects, is isotonic and pyrogen free and can be administered through a peripheral vein. The first fat preparations caused serious side effects—fever, coagulopathy and fat overload—probably due to the emulsifying agent, and they were withdrawn from use in 1965.[34] The authors suggested the feasibility of preparing a 10% fat, 5% amino acid and 3% glucose solution that could be given through a peripheral vein, though it is slightly hypertonic.

Potential complications of TPN are listed in Table 6–4. Although infection can be a serious complication of intravenous hyperalimentation, prevention is the key. Mixing individual sterilized components

TABLE 6-4.—POTENTIAL COMPLICATIONS OF TOTAL PARENTERAL NUTRITION

INFECTION AND SEPSIS	SUBCLAVIAN CATHETERIZATION	METABOLIC ALTERATIONS
Catheter entrance site	Pneumothorax	Glycosuria and osmotic diuresis
Contamination during insertion	Hemothorax	Hyperosmolar hyperglycemic dehydration
Long-term catheter placement	Hydrothorax	Hyperchloremic metabolic acidosis
Catheter seeding resulting from blood-borne infection or distant focus of infection	Tension pneumothorax	Electrolyte disturbances
Solution contamination	Subcutaneous emphysema	Hyper- and hyponatremia
	Brachial plexus injury	Hyper- and hypokalemia
	Subclavian artery injury	Hyper- and hypocalcemia
	Subclavian hematoma	Hypophosphatemia
	Central vein thrombophlebitis	Hypomagnesemia
	Arteriovenous fistula	Hyperammonemia
	Thoracic duct injury	Prerenal azotemia
	Hydromediastinum	Hyper- and hypovitaminosis A and D
	Air embolism	Liver function abnormalities
	Catheter embolism	Trace element deficiencies
	Catheter misplacement	Essential fatty acid deficiencies
	Cardiac perforation with tamponade	Congestive heart failure and pulmonary edema
	Endocarditis	

of the formula under a laminar flow hood in the hospital pharmacy minimizes contamination. Aseptic technique and good infection control procedures reduce the incidence of infection at the catheter site.[7] If the patient's laboratory values are carefully monitored, metabolic alterations may be detected and corrected before serious complications arise. Suggested laboratory studies to monitor patients on TPN are: (1) serum studies, including the measurement of electrolytes and glucose, daily in the initial stages of infusion and later at least three times a week; (2) weekly measurement of BUN, calcium, phosphate, proteins and magnesium; and (3) CBC at least once per week. Monitoring urine glucose is also important, with the goal of maintaining urine sugar 0 to 1+.

To evaluate whether or not the patient is receiving adequate nutrition, the following indicators are helpful: (1) weight gain, ¼ to ½ lb/ day; (2) fluid balance (to assure weight gain is tissue, not water); and (3) serum BUN and creatinine for monitoring nitrogen status (strive for positive nitrogen balance).[11, 12, 27] It also would seem appropriate to measure total serum protein and serum albumin weekly to assess the effectiveness of amino acid or protein therapy. Chen and his associates studied amino acid metabolism in parenteral nutrition. Their results revealed that use of amino acids for protein synthesis was directly proportional to the caloric supply (450 total cal = 1 gm nitrogen). Again, these investigators used BUN as a parameter of amino acid utilization during parenteral nutrition.[6]

In summary, the overall goal of total parenteral nutrition is to maintain an anabolic state and supply adequate quantities of essential nutrients.

CASE PRESENTATION.—R. G. is an 18-year-old man who was hospitalized because of an esophageal cutaneous fistula. The patient had undergone a small bowel resection at another hospital three months before this admission. The patient had had perforation of the mid-jejunum due to adhesions from a splenectomy and a partial left nephrectomy that had followed an auto accident at age 9. One of the adhesive bands had severed the jejunum. At that time, a high mid-jejunal jejunostomy was performed, and the distal ileum was closed. Ten days later, the patient developed pelvic abscesses that drained spontaneously into the rectum. The patient then underwent surgery to lyse adhesions, and a side-to-side jejunostomy was done. Following this, the patient developed severe upper GI bleeding; multiple stress ulcers were found; and the patient had a complete gastric resection. He was found at that time to have subdiaphragmatic abscesses. A tracheostomy was performed, and the patient did reasonably well. However, he developed a "spit" fistula from the distal end of the esophagus and several fistulas between the small bowel and the abdominal wall.

126 CLINICAL NUTRITION

During this period of time, the patient lost a considerable amount of weight and reached a low of 48 kg; his height was 175 cm. Purulent drainage from the fistula and drainage from the subdiaphragmatic abscess continued. He was then started on 3,000 ml hyperalimentation per day. The hyperalimentation contained Freamine II, 50% dextrose, 3.3 mM/L potassium phosphate, 40 mEq/L potassium chloride and 8.1 mEq/L magnesium sulfate. One of the three bottles contained 1 ampule MVI concentrated vitamins, and one bottle contained 100 mEq/L sodium chloride. The patient had parenteral hyperalimentation for a period of three months. His weight gradually increased and stabilized at 68 kg. The numerous small bowel fistulae, which had developed during the three-month period that the patient had been on dextrose and water and dextrose and saline only, gradually closed. The patient was then able to undergo a Roux-en-Y procedure to close the esophageal cutaneous fistula.

REFERENCES
1. Abbott, W. M., Abel, R. M., and Fischer, J. E.: The effects of total parenteral nutrition upon serum lipid levels, Surg. Gynecol. Obstet. 142:565, 1976.
2. Abel, R. M., et al.: Malnutrition in cardiac surgical patients, Arch. Surg. 111:45, 1976.
3. Bozzetti, F.: Parenteral nutrition in surgical patients, Surg. Gynecol. Obstet. 142:16, 1976.
4. Bradley, E. L., III, et al.: Nutritional consequences of total gastrectomy, Ann. Surg. 182:415, 1975.
5. Byrd, H. S., Lazarus, H. M., and Torma, M. J.: Effects of parenteral alimentation on postoperative gastric function, Am. J. Surg. 130:688, 1975.
6. Chen, W. J., Ohashi, E., and Kasai, M.: Amino acid metabolism in parenteral nutrition, with special reference to the calorie:nitrogen ratio and the blood urea nitrogen level, Metabolism 23:1117, 1974.
7. Copeland, E. M., MacFadyen, B. V., and Dudrick, S. J.: Prevention of microbial catheter contamination in patients receiving parenteral hyperalimentation, South. Med. J. 67:303, 1974.
8. Daly, J. M., et al.: Postoperative oral and intravenous nutrition, Ann. Surg. 180:709, 1974.
9. Driscoll, J. M., et al.: Total intravenous alimentation in low-birthweight infants: A preliminary report, J. Pediatr. 81:145, 1972.
10. Dudrick, S. J.: Intravenous hyperalimentation, Surgery 68:726, 1970.
11. Dudrick, S. J.: Total intravenous feeding, when nutrition seems impossible, Drug Ther. Bull. 1:11, 1976.
12. Dudrick, S. J., and Ruberg, R. L.: Principles and practice of parenteral nutrition, Gastroenterology 61:901, 1971.
13. Dudrick, S. J., et al.: Long-term total parenteral nutrition with growth, development and positive nitrogen balance, Surgery, 64:134, 1968.
14. Elwyn, D. H., Bryan-Brown, C. W., and Shoemaker, W. C.: Nutritional aspects of body water dislocations in postoperative and depleted patients, Ann. Surg. 182:76, 1975.
15. Feggetter, J. G.: Fat as a calorie source in parenteral nutrition (abstract), Proc. R. Soc. Med. 68:179, 1975.
16. Freeman, J. B., Egan, M. C., and Millis, B. J.: The elemental diet, Surg. Gynecol. Obstet. 142:925, 1976.

17. Jordan, G. L.: Surgical approach to nutritional problems, Adv. Surg. 8:85, 1974.
18. Kark, R. M.: Liquid formula and chemically defined diets, J. Am. Diet. Assoc. 64:476, 1974.
19. Manners, J. M.: Nutrition after cardiac surgery, Anaesthesia 29:675, 1974.
20. Mason, E. E., and Printen, K. J.: Metabolic considerations in reconstitution of the small intestine after jejunoileal bypass, Surg. Gynecol. Obstet. 142:177, 1976.
21. McKeown, K. C.: The surgical treatment of carcinoma of the esophagus, Proc. R. Soc. Med. 67:389, 1974.
22. Neviackas, J. A., and Kerstein, M. D.: Pancreatic enzyme response with an elemental diet, Surg. Gynecol. Obstet. 142:71, 1976.
23. Page, C. P., Ryan, J. A., and Hoff, R. C.: Continual catheter administration of an elemental diet, Surg. Gynecol. Obstet. 142:184, 1976.
24. Randall, H. T.: Diet and Nutrition in the Care of the Surgical Patient, in Goodhart, R. S., and Shils, M. E. (eds.): *Modern Nutrition in Health and Disease, Dietotherapy* (Philadelphia : Lea & Febiger, 1973).
25. Ross, W. M.: Radiotherapy of carcinoma of the esophagus, Proc. R. Soc. Med. 67:395, 1974.
26. Rutten, P., et al.: Determination of optimal hyperalimentation infusion rate, J. Surg. Res. 18:477, 1975.
27. Shils, M. E.: Total Parenteral Nutrition, in Goodhart, R. S., and Shils, M. E. (eds.): *Modern Nutrition in Health and Disease, Dietotherapy* (Philadelphia: Lea & Febiger, 1973).
28. Temple, W. J., et al.: Effect of nutrition, diet and suture material on long-term wound healing, Ann. Surg. 182:93, 1975.
29. Voitk, A. J.: The place of elemental diet in clinical nutrition, Br. J. Clin. Pract. 29:55, 1975.
30. Voitk, A. J., and Crispin, J. S.: The ability of an elemental diet to support nutrition and adaptation in the short gut syndrome, Ann. Surg. 181:220, 1975.
31. Walker, W. F.: Nutrition after injury, World Rev. Nutr. Diet. 19:173, 1973.
32. Wilmore, D. W.: Nutrition and metabolism following thermal injury, Clin. Plast. Surg. 1:603, 1974.
33. Wilson, J. P.: Postoperative motility of the large intestine in man, Gut 16:689, 1975.
34. Yeo, M. T., et al.: Total intravenous nutrition, experience with fat emulsions and hypertonic glucose, Arch. Surg. 106:792, 1973.
35. Young, E. A., et al.: Comparative nutritional analysis of chemically defined diets, Gastroenterology 69:1338, 1975.
36. Zohrab, W. J., McHattie, J. D., and Jeejeebhoy, K. N.: Total parenteral alimentation with lipid, Gastroenterology 64:583, 1973.

Chapter 7 / Nutrition and Diet Therapy in Renal Disease

DIETARY MANAGEMENT of patients with renal disease has been recognized as an effective method of treatment for over a decade. In the early 1960s, Giovannetti and Maggiore were the forerunners of the treatment of chronic uremia with a low nitrogen diet. Though theirs was a conservative approach, diet therapy is still of utmost importance for patients receiving peritoneal dialysis or hemodialysis for chronic renal failure. Often, the same or similar dietary modifications are made for patients in acute renal failure. The diet for patients with renal disease may be constantly changing, as the clinical situation and stage of the disease change. Dietary prescriptions are adjusted as the kidney's function diminishes.

The kidneys have three major functions: (1) excretion of the end products of protein metabolism—urea, uric acid, creatinine, organic acids and sulfate; (2) regulation of electrolyte and fluid balance—excretion and selective reabsorption of sodium, potassium, chloride and other ions plus water and selective excretion of excess acid to maintain acid-base equilibrium; and (3) endocrine production of renin, which acts on angiotensin to affect systémic blood pressure after release into the circulation, production of erythropoietin and conversion of inactive vitamin D after its initial hydroxylation in the liver to 1-25-dihydroxycholecalciferol, the biologically active metabolite.

Dietary treatment aims to (1) lighten the work of the diseased organ by reducing the amount of the excretory products; and (2) replace certain substances which are lost in abnormal amounts due to impaired renal function.[12]

Acute Renal Failure

Causes

According to Ogg, the most common cause of acute renal failure is acute tubular necrosis. Other possible causes are obstruction of both kidneys or of a solitary functioning kidney, acute glomerulonephritis, renal vascular occlusion, hemolytic uremic syndrome, renal cortical necrosis, acute pyelonephritis, acute interstitial nephritis, metabolic disorders, such as hypercalcemia or hyperuricemia, and leptospirosis.[54]

Treatment

For acute renal failure without hemodialysis in the oliguric phase, Mitchell and her associates and Jockes recommended the elimination of protein or its restriction to 10–20 gm/day.[51, 37] Sodium and potassium should be severely restricted, since the kidneys cannot filter them properly. If both these electrolytes are retained, they may approach lethal levels. Calories should be provided by oral infusions of glucose and carbohydrates that are low in sodium and potassium.[27] Total fluid intake should not exceed 500 ml (to replace insensible water loss from the skin and through the lungs) plus the volume of the previous day's urine output.[16]

Dialysis represents only a small fraction of the total treatment of these patients. Many patients with acute renal failure recover without this form of treatment. Timing of dialysis may be crucial and depend on overhydration, hyperkalemia, rate and direction of change in the clinical condition of the patient, blood or urine chemistry, associated medical and surgical problems and administrative problems. The aim of dialysis is to prevent the complications of renal failure, rather than to treat them after they arise.[54] Dialysis may have to be repeated several times before recovery.

In the early diuretic phase of acute renal failure, Jockes suggested a "light diet" without excess fluid and with sodium and potassium replaced quantitatively according to excretion. A "free diet" can be gradually introduced as kidney function returns to normal.[37]

Treatment of acute renal failure with intravenous administration of essential amino acids and glucose was studied by Abel and his associates. Sixteen (80%) of 20 patients who received a solution of 8 essential amino acids in 47% dextrose survived their episodes of acute renal failure, while 8 (40%) of 20 patients who received 50% dextrose solution survived. The solutions were administered via direct superior vena cava gravity infusion. Nine of the 16 surviving patients who received the essential amino acid solution did not require dialysis, in contrast to 6 similar patients who received the glucose solution. The improvement in patient survival and early recovery from acute renal failure in patients who received the essential amino acid solution suggested that the recovery of renal tubular function may be aided by the availability of essential amino acids and nitrogen as a substrate for protein synthesis.[1]

Glomerulonephritis presents a common problem in management of patients with acute renal failure and thus requires more extensive discussion. During the acute phase of renal failure, the ideal dietary content of protein and sodium is debatable. Lange stated that the diet should be protein-free and consist only of fruit juices fortified with sugar or dextrose to supply adequate calories. In addition, the sodium intake must be restricted to depress glomerular tubular imbalance.[42] Goodhart and Shils referred to the studies done in the late 1940s and early 1950s that supported the use of a regular to high protein intake, instead of a restricted protein intake, to prevent further tissue catabolism and promote the healing process. They claimed that salt should not be restricted unless hypertension, edema or oliguria were potential hazards.[28] The most sensible approach is to determine urinary loss of sodium while the patient is taking a known amount of dietary sodium. If undue sodium retention occurs, sodium should be restricted. Daily weighing of the patient also indicates whether sodium intake is too high.

Chronic Renal Failure

Causes

The most common causes of chronic renal failure are chronic glomerulonephritis, chronic pyelonephritis, hypertension, polycystic disease, analgesic nephropathy, obstructive uropathy, renal calculi, gout, diabetes mellitus, amyloidosis and collagen diseases, such as lupus erythematosus.[54, 12] The kidneys have a great reserve capacity and can maintain their excretory and regulatory capacity even if only 40% of the nephrons are functioning. When only 10% of the functioning kidney tissue remains, waste products of body metabolism accumulate in tissues and blood, since the kidneys are no longer able to excrete them adequately. Uremia develops, and death is imminent unless dialysis is initiated or renal transplantation is performed.

The uremic syndrome is characterized by retention of urea, creatinine and other products of protein metabolism in the blood and tissues, electrolyte disturbances, such as retention of potassium leading to hyperkalemia which induces cardiac arrhythmia and cardiac arrest, water retention and progressive acidosis. Anemia arises due to several factors: (1) toxic suppression of red blood cell production; (2) toxic shortening of the life span of erythrocytes; and (3) impaired production of erythropoietin by the nonfunctioning kidney. Serum phosphate is high, while calcium is low due to inhibition of intestinal absorption of calcium and the inability of kidneys to convert vitamin D into its active form.[12, 20, 22] However, rational dietary treatment can postpone dialysis for many months, depending on the rate of destruction of residual renal function.[12]

Objectives of Dietary Management

During the period before maintenance dialysis is required, conservative management is aimed at slowing the progression of the uremic syndrome.

CASE PRESENTATION.—A 46-year-old white male presented with blurred vision, fatigue and nausea. During the year prior to admission, he had taken an unknown "waterpill" but had not followed a sodium-restricted diet.

Past medical history was unremarkable, but the family history was positive for hypertension.

Physical examination revealed blood pressure 200/120 mm Hg, pulse 90 beats/min and respirations 16 resp/min. Funduscopic examination revealed clear discs, atrioventricular nicking, flame hemorrhages and waxy exudates. CV examination revealed S-4 but was otherwise unremarkable for the patient's age. Ischemic changes were shown on ECG, and the chest was within normal limits.

Laboratory examination showed BUN of 148 mg/dl, 8.1 mg/dl creatinine, 8.5 mg/dl calcium, 5.6 mg/dl phosphorus, 13.6 mg/dl uric acid, 4.3 mEq/L K^+. CBC showed hemoglobin 8.2 gm/dl, hematocrit 27%. Urinalysis revealed 4+ protein, 20–40 RBC/high power field and no red cell casts.

Hospital course: On admission, the patient was treated with intravenous antihypertensive medications to lower blood pressure. Medical evaluation during hospitalization was compatible with the diagnosis of chronic renal failure secondary to hypertension. At discharge, the patient was placed on a 20 gm, high-biologic value protein diet, with 60 mEq K^+, 1.5–2.0 gm Na^+ daily. Fluid restriction was 500 ml plus total urine output daily. Prescribed medications included 30 ml aluminum hydroxide gel by mouth before meals and one stool softener daily and $FeSO_4$, folic acid, vitamin B complex, furosemide (Lasix), propranolol, and hydralazine hydrochloride.

The patient's diet and fluid intake are manipulated so that residual renal function can be utilized as efficiently as possible.[54] As the residual renal function decreases, fluid and electrolyte balance can be maintained through careful monitoring of the patient's intake: Protein intake is restricted to 20–25 gm/day; 18–20 gm of the protein from sources of highest biologic value (e.g., eggs and milk). Sodium, potassium and phosphorus are restricted; fluid is restricted to the patient's output; and calories must be given in the form of special, synthetic, protein-free items (e.g., low protein noodles, rusks, cookies, cereal and puddings).

Progressive deterioration of renal function is accompanied by anor-

TABLE 7-1.—BURTON'S RECOMMENDATIONS
FOR DAILY DIETARY PROTEIN INTAKE
BASED ON CREATININE CLEARANCE[13]

CREATININE CLEARANCE (ML/MIN)	DAILY PROTEIN INTAKE (GM/DAY)
20-30	50
15-20	40
10-15	30
5-10	25

exia, nausea, vomiting and diarrhea and signals the need for protein restriction. Other clues to initiate adjustment of protein intake are creatinine clearance of less than 25 ml/min and BUN greater than 100 mg/dl. Burton recommended the schedule for adjusting daily protein intake shown in Table 7-1. Increments for urinary protein loss should be added to these amounts. Patients placed on chronic dialysis should receive 0.8-1.0 gm protein/kg body weight/day, since protein is lost through the dialysate.[12] Anderson described a slightly different approach for determining the appropriate protein intake: 0.5 gm protein/kg body weight/day if creatinine clearance is 20-30 ml/min; 0.38 gm protein/kg body weight/day if creatinine clearance is 5-19 ml/min; and 0.26 gm protein/kg body weight/day if creatinine clearance is less than 5 ml/min.[3]

Through repeated measurements of sodium and potassium in the serum and urine, desirable levels of sodium and potassium in the diet for renal patients may be determined. Sodium restriction is necessary to prevent sodium retention in the body, which leads to generalized edema. Likewise, hyperkalemia must be avoided to prevent cardiac arrhythmia and arrest. If either or both electrolytes are lost during severe vomiting or diarrhea, supplementation must be initiated carefully. Burton suggested a usual sodium intake of 500 mg daily and 250 mg sodium intake for an edematous patient unable to diurese with 500 mg.[12] However, Anderson stated that a less severe restriction of sodium, 40-90 mEq (1-2 gm) per day with the addition of furosemide would be adequate if the 40 mEq of sodium proved excessive. He did not feel that further reduction of sodium intake was practical. It should be remembered that patients with salt-losing nephritis require higher levels of sodium in the diet. If a patient appears to have normal total body sodium, the sodium prescription should be based on estimates of current sodium intake determined by a dietitian, if possible. The patient's sodium intake can be calculated by a rough estimate as follows: 90-100 mEq of sodium per day for patients who add no salt at the table and avoid salty foods and 200 mEg of sodium per day or more for patients who eat salty foods and salt foods generously before tasting.[3]

Fluid intake for patients with kidney failure must keep pace with the fluids eliminated from the body. Generally, the amount of fluid allowed is equal to the patient's 24-hour urine output plus 500–600 ml to replace insensible losses of water through the lungs, skin and feces. Burton advised an intake of 200–300 ml fluids more than the 24-hour urine output.[12]

Restriction of phosphate intake is encouraged to inhibit the development of secondary hyperparathyroidism. For patients on chronic dialysis who receive a fairly liberal protein intake, phosphate restriction becomes a greater problem. In this case, limiting the intake of milk and milk products high in phosphates is helpful. In addition, administration of aluminum hydroxide preparations acts to bind phosphates in the gut, thereby making them unabsorbable, and helps to control hyperphosphatemia.[12]

Vitamin supplementation is advisable when there is a prolonged, severe protein restriction. This is due to the fact that so many foods must be eliminated from a diet restricted to 40 gm protein or less. Also, patients on dialysis must be given multiple vitamins daily, since there is considerable loss of water-soluble vitamins from the blood during dialysis.[12]

Calories should not be restricted in the diet for a patient with renal failure. An adequate supply of carbohydrates and fats spares protein and prevents tissue catabolism. To achieve a caloric intake of 2,000–3,000 kcal with a protein-restricted diet and reduced sodium and potassium is a challenge for the dietitian who plans the diet and for the patient who consumes it. Cost reviewed the importance of kilocalories in the diet for patients with chronic renal disease. There are only 1,400 kcal in the usual 50 gm protein, 2 gm sodium, and 2 gm potassium diet. However, she demonstrated how the caloric intake could be increased by using recipes high in calories and low in protein. These foods could be substituted for servings of foods allowed on the food lists. For example, a dessert, such as low protein apple cake, containing 2 gm protein and 225 kcal, can be substituted for one slice of bread, which contains 2 gm protein but only 70 kcal.[17]

Chronic Glomerulonephritis and Nephrosclerosis

The clinical course of chronic glomerulonephritis may demonstrate a prolonged latent stage, followed by a nephrotic stage and then renal insufficiency with nitrogen retention or uremia. For patients with moderate renal insufficiency in the chronic phase of glomerulonephritis, Lange suggests a protein intake of more than 30 gm *as long as* there is no marked elevation in BUN. When the glomerular filtration rate falls to 10 mg/min or below and serum creatinine values rise above 6 mg/dl, more stringent dietary restrictions, as for patients with chronic renal failure, become necessary.[42] Dietary protein is restricted to 45–65 gm/day as the BUN begins to rise. Calories are given liberally in the form of carbohydrates and fats. Further decreases in the daily protein allowance will be needed as the BUN continues to climb. The sodium restriction required in the nephrotic stage is revoked, since the kidneys are unable to conserve sodium and chloride. Fluid intake should be kept between 2,500 and 3,500 ml daily for proper renal clearance of nitrogenous wastes, as long as the failing kidneys waste salt and cardiac function is not impaired. Dietary management in acute, malignant nephrosclerosis is the same as described above.[13]

The Nephrotic Syndrome

This syndrome exhibits albuminuria, hypoalbuminemia, hypercholesterolemia and massive edema and may be seen during the nephrotic stage of chronic glomerulonephritis, in lupus nephritis, lipoid nephrosis, renal amyloidosis and other disorders. The kidneys' inability to excrete salt normally leads to salt retention and consequently to edema, which compounds the effects of hypoalbuminemia. Diet therapy seeks a high protein intake and severe sodium restriction. Protein intake must be high enough to compensate for urinary loss and encourage synthesis of plasma albumin. Daily protein intake will vary from 95 to 130 gm, depending on the patient's weight and urinary protein loss. Burton recommended sodium restriction of 500 mg or less due to the patient's sodium retention. With such a strict sodium intake, fluids may be allowed freely.[13]

Advanced Renal Failure without Dialysis

When the glomerular filtration rate drops to about 10 ml/min, the patient's diet must be adjusted quite markedly to prevent retention of metabolic waste products and end-stage uremia. If, for some reason, the patient cannot undergo dialysis or transplantation, a special diet can prolong life and eliminate symptoms of advanced uremia for many months. However, a glomerular filtration rate of 2–3 ml/min is required for patients to survive on this diet. The principles of this diet are minimum protein in the form of essential amino acids (high-biologic value protein) to maintain nitrogen balance, along with abundant calories in the form of unlimited carbohydrates and fats, which do not require the kidneys to remove metabolic waste products. The body can thereby synthesize necessary nonessential amino acids by using pathologically overabundant urea in blood and tissue. These are the same principles upon which Giordano and Giovannetti based their diet in the early 1960s.[27]

The Giordano-Giovannetti diet supplies about 20 gm of protein/day of high biologic value. The daily allowance includes one egg and ¾ cup of milk. Occasionally, the egg may be replaced by 1 oz of meat, fish or poultry. The diet supplies 2,000–3,000 kcal, mostly carbohydrates (wheat starch products) and fats. Low protein bread and pastas are commercially available, and recipes using wheat starches are given to patients. In addition, low protein, low potassium fruits and vegetables (Table 7–2) are added to the diet, along with unlimited quantities of sugars and fats.[25-27] Others have made modifications to this particular diet, but all have used the same principles.[10, 41, 47, 70, 76] Fluid intake is limited to the usual level of lung, skin and stool losses plus urine output, if any.[16, 46, 76] Sodium intake may vary from 500 to 2,000 mg; potassium may vary from 1,500 to 2,300 mg.

Obviously, the success of this life-maintaining diet depends on the patient's strict adherence to a very restrictive diet. Consumption of

TABLE 7–2.—FRUITS AND VEGETABLES
LOW IN POTASSIUM*

	SERVING (GM)
Apple, fresh	90
Apple juice	100
Applesauce	100
Cherries, canned or frozen	75
Cranberry juice cocktail	480
Grape juice, frozen	100
Pears, canned	100
Pineapple, canned or frozen	100
Strawberries, frozen, whole, sweetened	100
Watermelon, fresh	100
Beans, green or wax, canned	100
Carrots, canned	100
Corn, canned	100
Cucumbers, fresh	50
Lettuce, fresh	45
Peas, canned	100
Pepper, fresh, green	40
Sweet potatoes, canned in syrup	100

*100–120 mg K+ per serving

the entire number of calories prescribed to prevent tissue catabolism is also of utmost importance. Use of the many special foods available for treating chronic renal failure will assure adequate caloric intake. Karp described the many uses of electrodialyzed whey, from milk-like beverages to desserts and spreads.[40] Smith reported the use of wheat starch in making protein-free bread.[67] Other commercially available products are low protein pastas, such as cereal, noodles and macaroni; low protein rusks; low protein, high calorie drinks; and a low protein, low sodium milk substitute.

The importance of adequate caloric intake cannot be stressed enough. To demonstrate what happens when caloric levels are inadequate, Betts and Magrath studied the growth pattern of children with chronic renal insufficiency. They noted that the development of impaired renal function in infancy had a more damaging effect on linear growth than did onset in later years. Reduction in rate of growth was found when the glomerular filtration rate fell below 25 ml/min/1.73 M. Children with renal insufficiency had a significantly reduced intake of calories, protein and vitamin D in comparison to the recommended amounts for their age. Their caloric intake was significantly reduced when compared with that of normal children of their own height. Reduced growth rate occurred when caloric intake fell below 80% of the recommended level.[9] Simmons reported similar results when children on hemodialysis received less than 70% of the RDA for kcal.[65]

When a patient is no longer able to excrete urea in sufficient quantities to balance his restricted protein intake, dialysis and a diet much more generous than that followed during conservative management are required.

Advanced Renal Failure with Dialysis

When the glomerular filtration rate falls to 1.5 ml/min, dialysis with an artificial kidney is required to remove metabolic waste products and alleviate symptoms of uremia. In contrast to the severely restricted diet a patient must follow under conservative management, the diet for patients on dialysis is very liberal. Diet becomes very important in determining biochemical control after initiation of maintenance dialysis for patients who have lost all renal function. The aim of diet therapy is to administer the quantity of protein, sodium, potassium and fluids that can be held in equilibrium by dialysis.[46, 13]

CASE PRESENTATION.—A 42-year-old white male presented with a two-week history of nausea and vomiting, increasing lethargy and swelling of ankles, hands and face. Twenty years prior to admission, he was told that he had "nephritis" and that he might gradually lose kidney function.

Physical examination revealed blood pressure 160/105 mm Hg, pulse 90 beats/min and respiration 18 resp/min. The patient's skin was pale, and eyelids were puffy. CV examination showed S-3 and S-4 and pericardial friction rub. The extremities showed 2+ edema, pretibial.

Laboratory examination included BUN 220 mg/dl, 23 mg/dl creatinine, 6.8 mEq/L K+, pH 7.15.

Hospital course: Peritoneal dialysis was initiated in the first hours after admission, and the patient's symptoms and laboratory results showed gradual improvement. Evaluation suggested that chronic renal failure was secondary to chronic glomerulonephritis and that the patient was a candidate for chronic hemodialysis. He was discharged to return for dialysis three times weekly. Upon discharge, the patient was placed on a diet of 60 gm high-biologic value protein (1 gm/kg), 60–80 mEq K+, and 2 gm Na+. Fluid restriction was 500 ml plus daily urine output. Discharge medications included aluminum hydroxide gel, a stool softener, ferrous sulfate, folic acid, vitamin B-complex and pyridoxine.

The protein allowance is somewhat variable according to which source is quoted. Mayer stated 0.5–0.6 gm/kg ideal weight was adequate, but he also stated that 1 gm/kg ideal weight was safer.[48] Mackenzie recommended 0.8–1.0 gm/kg ideal weight.[46] Burton suggested that a protein allowance of 1 gm/kg ideal weight would *not* result in the buildup of excessive nitrogenous waste products. This amount would replace those amino acids lost through dialysis and would maintain positive nitrogen balance.[13]

Sodium intake varies according to the severity of hypertension and edema. Mackenzie suggested that sodium intake might be as high as 2,000 mg rather than the very low 500 mg others have used.[46] According to Burton, 65–87 mEq (1,500–2,000 mg) of sodium daily will control fluid retention and hypertension and will not interfere with the patient's appetite or the diet's palatability.[13] Patients must learn to read all labels carefully to avoid intake of excessive amounts of sodium. Commercially prepared products are eliminated from the diet because of their salt content. Salt substitutes cannot be used because of their potassium content.

Potassium should be restricted if hyperkalemia is present. Hyperkalemia can result in cardiac arrhythmias or arrest with little or no warning. Therefore, frequent checks on the patient's serum potassium level are essential for cautious monitoring of dietary potassium. Generally, 1–2 gm potassium/day is the daily diet order (mEq = 39 mg). Burton suggested 52 mEq potassium daily for a dialysate bath containing 2.6 mEq potassium.[13] Potassium restriction is difficult due to the high amounts present in meat, milk and many fruits and vegetables

TABLE 7-3.—FOODS HIGH IN POTASSIUM

FOOD	SERVING	K+ CONTENT (MG/SERVING)
Banana, fresh	1 medium	628
Beans, kidney	100 gm	1,310
Beans, lima	100 gm	680
Beets, tops	100 gm	570
Bread, pumpernickel	1 slice	454
Broccoli	100 gm	400
Brussels sprouts	100 gm	450
Cauliflower, cooked	100 gm	400
Cauliflower, raw	1¼ cup	500
Chocolate, milk, sweetened	1 cup	420
Chocolate, plain, sweetened	100 gm	397
Cocoa, dry powder	100 gm	900–3,200
Dandelion greens	100 gm	430
Dates, dried	100 gm	790
Figs, dried	7 small	780
Fruit cocktail, canned	1 cup	410
Grapefruit juice, canned	1 cup	405
Kale	100 gm	410
Lentils, dried	100 gm	810
Molasses	100 gm	1,500
Mushrooms	100 gm	520
Nuts	100 gm	147–972 (depending on kind)
Orange juice, fresh	1 cup	496
Peaches, dried	½ cup	1,100
Peanut butter	100 gm	670
Peas, dried, split	100 gm	880
Potato chips	100 gm	880
Potatoes, raw	100 gm	410
Prunes, dried, uncooked	100 gm	700
Prune juice, canned	1 cup	563
Raisins, dried	100 gm	725
Salt substitutes	1 gm	~450
Spinach, fresh	100 gm	662
Sweetbreads	100 gm	519
Sweet potatoes	100 gm	530
Swiss chard	100 gm	550
Tomato juice, canned	1 cup	544
Turnip greens	100 gm	440
Wheat germ	100 gm	737

(Table 7-3). Vitamins, calories and protein are essential for proper nutrition.

Fluids should be restricted to a total equal to the patient's urine output, if any, plus an amount to cover insensible losses in a 24-hour period. Mackenzie stated that most oliguric or anuric hypertensive patients require fluid restriction of 300–500 ml plus an amount equal to urinary output. He suggested that, in addition to the prescribed fluid, fluids in foods and water from catabolism of food would result in a daily weight gain of 1 lb (mild fluid retention) between periods of dialysis.[46]

Calories to prevent tissue breakdown are supplied through generous amounts of low protein carbohydrates and fats. A prescription of 35–45 kcal/kg ideal body weight is usually recommended; 45 kcal/kg are especially important for weight gain and tissue building.[13]

Again, it is suggested that a multiple vitamin tablet and iron supplement be prescribed to replace nutrients lost in dialysis. This is especially true of ascorbic acid and folic acid.[13]

A diet therapy program and the educational materials developed for patients at the Public Health Service Hospital in San Francisco were described by Robinson and Paulbitski a few years ago. Composition of diets for patients on renal dialysis and samples of the selective menus were presented in their report. Individualization and variety of diets were stressed. A programmed instruction booklet with recipes was developed to help patients control their intake of restricted nutrients.[62] Stein and Winn presented a different approach to the patient's freedom of choice in food selection and dietary education. Use of "points" for dietary calculation of protein, sodium and potassium was developed and initiated at the University of Kansas Medical Center. One "point" represented one unit of food value, such as 1 mEq of sodium or potassium and 1 gm of protein. A booklet listed foods by groups showing sodium, potassium and protein points for each item.[71]

Vetter and Shapiro at the Medical College of Ohio described an approach to dietary management of patients with renal disease in which diet palatability and patient education are the main objectives. Again, lists of allowed foods were accompanied by lists of alternate foods of similar protein, sodium and potassium content. The number of servings from each list was determined by the diet prescription. Instruction in diet and recipe preparation was initiated soon after the diet was ordered. A three-week selective cycle menu was developed as a teaching tool and allowed more variety.[74]

Development of hypertriglyceridemia secondary to chronic renal failure has been reported by Bagdade and others.[5] McCosh and her associates studied the development of hypertriglyceridemia in 38 patients with chronic renal insufficiency.[49] Patients in moderate and severe stages of chronic renal insufficiency showed significantly elevated plasma triglycerides. Patients on chronic hemodialysis had a further increase in plasma triglycerides. Prior to hemodialysis, serum electrophoretic studies revealed elevated chylomicrons and very low-density lipoprotein fractions. Hyperchylomicronemia predominated in patients on chronic hemodialysis.[49]

Calcium, Phosphorus and Vitamin D in Uremia

Dietary management of patients with chronic renal failure must consider reducing the incidence of bone lesions from secondary hyperparathyroidism and osteomalacia. Osteitis fibrosa cystica, osteomalacia, osteopenia, osteosclerosis and metastatic calcification have been referred to as renal osteodystrophy in patients with chronic renal disease. Since the advent of chronic dialysis therapy, renal osteodystrophy and disturbed divalent ion metabolism have been researched and have led to better understanding of the pathogenesis of uremic bone disease.[64] Control of serum phosphate levels and positive calcium balance are the most important factors in treating osteodystrophy. The elegant work of Slatopolsky has greatly expanded our understanding of the sequence of events leading to the development of secondary hyperparathyroidism in chronic renal disease. His study in dogs showed that as glomerular filtration decreases and serum phosphorus begins to rise, there is a fall in the ionized serum calcium level, which leads to stimulation of the parathyroid glands and a consequent rise in serum parathyroid hormone concentration.[66]

Abnormalities in vitamin D metabolism further complicate the problem of calcium and phosphorus regulation. The 1-hydroxylation of 25-hydroxycholecalciferol by the kidney becomes impaired, both because of a decreased number of renal cells capable of metabolism and because of the high serum phosphorus levels that tend to induce 24-hydroxylation rather than 1-hydroxylation. In the absence of the active metabolite, 1-25-dihydroxycholecalciferol, calcium absorption

Fig 7–1.—Renal failure.

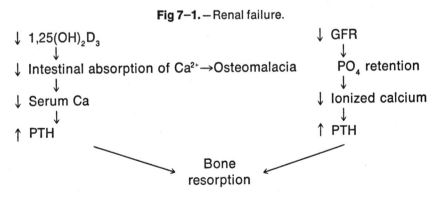

from the intestine is markedly impaired and results in further lowering of the serum ionized calcium level, which stimulates the parathyroid glands (Fig 7–1). The combination of defective vitamin D metabolism and hyperparathyroidism can result in bone diseases ranging from osteomalacia to osteitis fibrosa cystica.

Popovtzer and his associates reported that use of phosphate-binding antacids and calcium carbonate to maintain serum calcium at 9 mg/dl and serum phosphorus at 3.5 mg/dl resulted in the disappearance of symptoms of secondary hyperparathyroidism.[60] The new, experimental vitamin D preparations 1α-hydroxy vitamin D_3, 1-25-dihydroxy vitamin D, 5-6-*trans* vitamin D_3 and the currently available preparation dihydrotachysterol may improve calcium absorption from the intestine and decrease the incidence of severe secondary hyperparathyroidism.[20]

Restriction of phosphorus intake is important also in controlling the calcium-phosphorus product to prevent extraosseous calcification.[60] Providing a low phosphorus diet is very difficult in the face of increasing the calcium intake and supplying adequate protein, since meat and milk products are high in all three of these nutrients. At best, milk intake can be severely restricted. It must be kept in mind that, if followed for an extended period of time, a low phosphorus diet could result in phosphate depletion and further bone demineralization.

Renal Stones

One of the oldest recognized maladies in man is renal stones. It is estimated that, in the United States, renal stones account for one of every 1,000 hospitalizations, or approximately 200,000 hospitalized patients per year. In this country, 2/3 of all renal stones are composed of either calcium oxalate or calcium oxalate mixed with phosphate in the form of hydroxyapatite. Pure calcium phosphate stones are very rare. Fifteen percent of the stones are composed of magnesium ammonium phosphate, and these occur almost exclusively in patients with recurrent urinary tract infections, with urea-splitting organisms resulting in persistently alkaline urine. Uric acid and cystine stones together account for about 10%, and 9% are accounted for by a miscellaneous category including xanthine, silicate or matrix stones.[78]

Three major theories have been proposed to explain stone formation and growth: (1) the precipitation-crystallization theory; (2) the matrix nucleation theory; and (3) the inhibitor absence theory. The precipitation theory implies that supersaturation of urinary crystalloids eventually leads to their precipitation. This mechanism is most likely to be involved in the formation of stones composed of cystine, uric acid, xanthine and mixed magnesium-ammonium-phosphate stones. The matrix nucleation theory is based on the idea that some matrix substance forms an initial nucleus, and subsequent stones are formed by precipitation. Pak has presented data to suggest that calcium phosphate monohydrate functions as a nucleus for calcium oxalate stones.[55] Boyce has suggested that a urinary microprotein or uric acid may play this role.[11] Supporters of the inhibitor absence theory have pointed out that normal urine can hold larger amounts of crystalloids in solution than can simple aqueous solutions. It is proposed that normal urine therefore contains inhibitors of crystal formation and that the urine of stone formers does not contain these inhibitors.[52] A number of pertinent inhibitors of crystal formation have been identified in normal urine, including pyrophosphate, small polypeptides, urea, citrate, magnesium mucopolysaccharides, diphosphonates, trace metals and certain amino acids.

Patients with renal calculi should be evaluated to determine whether or not any metabolic abnormality is present. Despite the proposal of the three pathogenic mechanisms just described, the study of patients with recurrent stone disease generally involves a search for increased secretion of specific urinary crystalloids, particularly calcium, oxalate, uric acid, cystine and ammonia. The best understood forms of stone disease are those associated with hypercalcuria, hyperoxaluria, hyperuricuria, cystinuria and increased excretion of magnesium-ammonium-phosphate. However, it must be kept in mind that in the vast majority of patients who develop renal calculi, no metabolic abnormalities can be found. These patients fall into the idiopathic category.

For a patient with calcium stones, it is very important to determine whether or not he has hypercalcuria. Nordin defines it as urinary excretion of calcium of more than 300 mg/day for males or 250 mg/day for females.[53] As already mentioned, most of the patients with calcium stones have normal urinary excretion of calcium, but when hypercalcuria is present, it can be divided into three major categories: (1) resorptive hypercalcuria (hyperparathyroidism); (2) absorptive hypercalcuria; and (3) renal hypercalcuria. Differentiation of the type of hypercalcuria is important, since treatment depends upon the cause of the hypercalcuria. Pak has recently described a test that is helpful in distinguishing these three causes.[56] The essential steps in the test are to measure the ratio of calcium to creatinine and cyclic adenosine monophosphate excretion in the urine in the fasting state and then after an oral calcium load. The anticipated results are shown in Table 7–4.

TABLE 7–4.—PAK TEST FOR HYPERCALCURIA

	FASTING URINE CA/CR	POST-CA LOAD URINE CA/CR	FASTING cAMP	POST-CA cAMP
Normal	<0.11	<0.13	Normal	Decreased
Resorptive	>0.11	>0.2	Normal or high	High
Absorptive	<0.11	>0.2	Low or normal	Low or normal
Renal	>0.11	>0.13	High	Decreased

This table shows urinary calcium/mg creatinine and urinary cAMP/gm creatinine after a 12-hour fast and 4 hours after 1 gm oral calcium load.

This test will require further evaluation before we will know how accurate it is in separating the groups of hypercalcuria, but at present, it appears promising. From a therapeutic standpoint, this separation is exceedingly important, since restriction of dietary calcium should be reserved only for those patients with absorptive hypercalcuria. Nordin has shown that small reductions in dietary calcium may increase the absorption of oxalate.[53] Small increases in urinary oxalate concentrations augment the propensity for stone formation more markedly than do increases in urine calcium.

For patients with idiopathic hypercalcuria (absorptive hypercalcuria), dietary restriction of calcium is beneficial. Treatment is usually initiated with a diet containing 400 mg calcium per day. It is important then to repeat the 24-hour urine collection to determine whether or not the treatment is beneficial. In addition to calcium restriction, there are favorable reports of treatment using phosphogel as a binding agent to reduce the gastrointestinal absorption of calcium.[55]

The treatment of hyperparathyroidism is obvious, i.e., removal of the parathyroid adenoma. For patients with renal hypercalcuria, it has been shown that thiazide diuretics may be of benefit, since they increase the tubular reabsorption of calcium.[39]

Several other dietary correlations have been made. Phillips and Cooke demonstrated a relationship between calcium and sodium excretion in individuals with normal plasma sodium and calcium.[58] High levels of urinary calcium excretion were found in association with high levels of sodium excretion. Dietary restriction of sodium, resulting in decreased urinary sodium, was accompanied by a decrease in urinary calcium. This was found to be particularly helpful for paraplegics with hypercalcuria due to immobilization. When these patients were placed on a low salt diet (1 gm of sodium chloride/day) and a thiazide diuretic, they showed a 58% reduction in urinary excretion of sodium and a 53% reduction in urinary calcium excretion.[30] Sodium restriction appears to be safe and often very effective in the management of hypercalcuria.

Several efforts have been made to increase the urinary excretion of inhibitors of calcium precipitation. Fleisch et al. proposed the use of inorganic orthophosphate to induce an increase in urinary inorganic pyrophosphate.[24] The administration of phosphate is coming into disfavor because it induces secondary hyperparathyroidism.[38] Diphosphonates have also been suggested, since they, too, inhibit crystal formation. Increase in urinary magnesium after oral magnesium supplementation also appears to inhibit precipitation of calcium salts.

Hyperoxaluria must also be considered in patients with calcium oxalate stones, and urinary oxalate levels should be measured. The normal amount of oxalate in the urine is 50–60 mg/24 hours. Six major causes of hyperoxaluria have been identified in man: (1) increased ingestion of oxalate or precursors; (2) pyridoxine deficiency; (3) primary hyperoxaluria type I; (4) primary hyperoxaluria type II; (5) methoxyflurane anesthesia; and (6) hyperoxaluria secondary to ileal disease. Oxalic acid is a common organic acid found in many green, leafy vegetables, but these are not usually absorbed efficiently from the gastrointestinal tract in the normal person. Oxalate is also a metabolic end product in man derived from glyoxylic acid, its immediate precursor. Some urinary oxalate may also be derived from ascorbic acid. Hyperoxaluria has been reported from diets extremely high in oxalate (rhubarb poisoning), and it has been noted to occur after the ingestion of ethylene glycol contained in antifreeze. Since pyridoxine is an important cofactor in the transamination of glyoxalate to glycine, deficiency of this vitamin may lead to glyoxalate accumulation, with subsequent oxidation to oxalate.

Kaplan and Pak recommend dietary restriction of oxalate if hyperoxaluria is actually documented.[39] Foods high in oxalate are listed in Table 7–5. In addition, high doses of vitamin B_6 are recommended to decrease oxalate excretion. Other authorities have felt that the low oxalate diet is very ineffective and instead have recommended treatment with magnesium oxide, pyridoxine supplements and increased phosphate intake.[61] Protein restriction is not successful in sufficiently reducing glycine to prevent oxalate synthesis.

Gutman and Yu suggested that uric acid stone formation could be reduced by decreasing protein intake to less than 90 gm/day, administering allopurinol to inhibit synthesis of uric acid and increasing fluid intake, especially in the evenings, to increase solubility. They did not feel that the avoidance of purine-rich foods was so important because

TABLE 7-5.—FOODS HIGH
IN OXALATE

	OXALATE VALUES (MG/100 GM FOOD)
Beets, peeled	338
Beets, tops	916
Cocoa, dry powder	450
Rhubarb	230-500
Spinach, fresh	460
Spinach, canned	364
Swiss chard	690

Other high oxalate foods are asparagus, chocolate, cranberries, dandelion greens, some varieties of nuts and wheat germ.

of the advent of allopurinol.[31] Kaplan and Pak suggested the use of sodium citrate or bicarbonate to alkalinize the urine of these patients.[39]

Cystinuria is a rather rare disorder resulting in stone formation and this is discussed in more detail in Chapter 4.

In the control or treatment of renal calculi from any cause, increase in the urine volume by the administration of large amounts of fluid is extremely important. Dent recommended the establishment of diuresis to avoid supersaturated urine in the early morning hours. In addition to daytime water intake (500 ml every four hours), patients were instructed to drink two glasses of water at bedtime and two glasses at 2 A.M. This is particularly important to control stones that are due mainly to supersaturation, such as cystine and uric acid stones, and has been shown to decrease the incidence of stone formation.[21]

Therapy for renal stones is difficult to evaluate with accuracy because it takes many years to observe its effect. Ettinger pointed out that the effect of any form of therapy for calculi must be compared with the approximately 50% reduction in stone passage that is found during 2-3 years observation with placebo.[23]

Formation of Council on Renal Nutrition

The Council on Renal Nutrition was founded in 1974 as an advisory council to the National Kidney Foundation on issues concerning renal nutrition. The first annual meeting to review current practices and research in dietary management of patients with renal failure was held November 15 and 16, 1974, in San Francisco. The second meeting was held November 21 and 22, 1975, in New York City.

The objectives of the Council of Renal Nutrition are: (1) to develop and distribute information on the nutritional aspects of renal disease, dialysis, transplantation and other related disorders; (2) to develop and promote continuing education programs; (3) to promote legislation concerning related nutritional problems; and (4) to establish better nutritional care of patients through liaison with other professional organizations, develop endorsement critiques and publish position papers.[72]

REFERENCES

1. Abel, R. M., et al.: Treatment of acute renal failure with intravenous administration of essential amino acids and glucose, Surg. Forum 23:77, 1972.
2. Adlin, E. V., Biddle, C. M., and Channick, B. J.: Hypertensive patients with normal and low plasma renin activity, Am. J. Med. Sci. 261:67, 1971.
3. Anderson, C. F.: Treatment of chronic renal failure, Minn. Med. 57:364, 1974.
4. Arneil, G. C.: The nephrotic syndrome, Pediatr. Clin. North Am. 18:547, 1971.
5. Bagdade, J. D., and Bierman, E. L.: Diagnosis and dietary treatment of blood lipid disorders, Med. Clin. North Am. 54:1383, 1970.
6. Berlyne, G. M., and Epstein, N.: Dialysed milk in low-sodium and low-potassium diets for renal, hepatic and cardiac disease, Lancet 2:24, 1971.
7. Berlyne, G. M., Gaan, D., and Graks, W. R.: Dietary treatment of chronic renal failure, Am. J. Clin. Nutr. 21:547, 1968.
8. Berlyn, G. M., and Shaw, A. B.: Giordano-Giovannetti diet in terminal renal failure, Lancet 2:7, 1965.
9. Betts, P. R., and Magrath, G.: Growth patterns and dietary intake of children with chronic renal insufficiency, Br. Med. J. 2:189, 1974.
10. Blainey, J. D., and Chamberlain, M. J.: Dietary treatment of chronic renal failure, Br. Med. Bull. 27:160, 1971.
11. Boyce, W. H.: Organic matrix of human urinary concretions, Am. J. Med. 45:673, 1968.
12. Burton, B. T.: Current concepts of nutrition and diet in diseases of the kidney, I. General principles of dietary management, J. Am. Diet. Assoc. 65:623, 1974.
13. Burton, B. T.: Current concepts of nutrition and diet in diseases of the kidney, II. Dietary regimen in specific kidney disorders, J. Am. Diet. Assoc. 65:627, 1974.
14. Burton, B. T.: Diet therapy in uremia, J. Am. Diet. Assoc. 54:475, 1969.
15. Carmena, R., and Shapiro, F. L.: Dietary management of chronic renal failure: Experience at Hennepin County General Hospital, Geriatrics 27:95, 1972.
16. Clark, J. E., and Caedo, R. E.: Fluid and electrolyte management in renal failure, Am. Fam. Physician 5:124, 1972.
17. Cost, J. S.: Diet in chronic renal disease: A focus on calories, J. Am. Diet. Assoc. 64:186, 1974.
18. Crawhall, J. C., and Watts, R. W. E.: Cystinuria, Am. J. Med. 45:736, 1968.

19. Cullen, A. B.: Dietary management of chronic uremia and patient adherence to dietary restriction, Am. J. Clin. Nutr. 21:626, 1968.
20. David, D. S.: Calcium metabolism in renal failure, Am. J. Med. 58:48, 1975.
21. Dent, C. E., and Senior, B.: Studies in the treatment of cystinuria, Br. J. Urol. 27:317, 1955.
22. Epstein, F. H.: Calcium and the kidney, Am. J. Med. 45:700, 1968.
23. Ettinger, B.: Recurrent nephrolithiasis: Natural history and effect of phosphate therapy, Am. J. Med. 61:200, 1976.
24. Fleisch, H., Bisaz, S., and Care, A. D.: Effect of orthophosphate on urinary pyrophosphate excretion and the prevention of urolithiasis, Lancet 1:1065, 1964.
25. Giordano, C., et al.: Use of different sources of nitrogen in uremia, Arch. Intern. Med. 126:787, 1970.
26. Giovannetti, S., et al.: Implications of dietary therapy, Arch. Intern. Med. 126:900, 1970.
27. Giovannetti, S., and Maggiore, Q.: A low-nitrogen diet with proteins of high biological value for severe chronic uremia, Lancet 1:1000, 1964.
28. Goodhart, R. S., and Shils, M. E.: *Modern Nutrition in Health and Disease, Dietotherapy* (5th ed.; Philadelphia: Lea & Febiger, 1973), p. 852.
29. Gordon, R. D., et al.: Hypertension and severe hyperkalemia associated with suppression of renin and aldosterone and completely reversed by dietary sodium restriction, Aust. Ann. Med. 19:287, 1970.
30. Griffith, D. P.: Control of hypercalcuria in the immobilized patient, J. Urol. 105:698, 1971.
31. Gutman, A. B., and Yu, T. F.: Uric acid nephrolithiasis, Am. J. Med. 45: 756, 1968.
32. Hedger, R. W.: The conservative management of acute oliguric renal failure, Med. Clin. North Am. 55:121, 1971.
33. Holliday, M. A., Potter, D. E., and Dobrin, R. S.: Treatment of renal failure in children, Pediatr. Clin. North Am. 18:613, 1971.
34. Holmes, J. H.: The physician's responsibility in management of food and fluid intake, Trans. Am. Clin. Climatol. Assoc. 80:137, 1969.
35. Howard, J. E., and Thomas, W. C., Jr.: Control of crystallization in urine, Am. J. Med. 45:693, 1968.
36. Hunt, J. C., et al.: Renal and renovascular hypertension, Arch. Intern. Med. 133:988, 1974.
37. Jockes, A. M.: Conservative management of acute reversible renal failure, J. Irish Med. Assoc. 64:446, 1971.
38. Jowsey, J., Reiss, E., and Canterbury, J. M.: Long-term effect of high phosphate intake on parathyroid hormone levels and bone metabolism, Acta Orthop. Scand. 45:801, 1974.
39. Kaplan, R. A., and Pak, C. Y. C.: Diagnosis and management of renal calculi, Tex. Med. 70:88, 1974.
40. Karp, N. R.: Electrodialyzed whey-based foods for use in chronic uremia, J. Am. Diet. Assoc. 59:568, 1971.
41. Kopple, J. D., et al.: Controlled comparison of 20-g and 40-g protein diets in the treatment of chronic uremia, Am. J. Clin. Nutr. 21:553, 1968.
42. Lange, K.: Nutritional management of kidney disorders, Med. Clin. North Am. 55:513, 1971.
43. Leenen, F. H.: Relationships of the renin-angiotensin-aldosterone system

and sodium balance to blood pressure regulation in chronic renal failure of polycystic kidney disease, Metabolism 24:589, 1975.
44. Levin, M. L.: Food for thought in chronic renal disease, South. Med. J. 64:90, 1971.
45. Lindeman, R. D.: Influence of various nutrients and hormones on urinary divalent cation excretion, Ann. N.Y. Acad. Sci. 162:802, 1969.
46. Mackenzie, J. C.: Nutrition and dialysis, World Rev. Nutr. Diet. 13:194, 1971.
47. Matter, B. J.: Diet therapy of uremia, J. Okla. State Med. Assoc. 64:445, 1971.
48. Mayer, J.: Diet and renal disease, Postgrad. Med. 49:241, 1971.
49. McCosh, E. J., et al.: Hypertriglyceridemia in patients with chronic renal insufficiency, Am. J. Clin. Nutr. 28:1036, 1975.
50. Mehbod, H., Baskin, M., and Moss, J.: Diet in uremia, Am. Fam. Physician 4:75, 1971.
51. Mitchell, H. S., et al.: *Cooper's Nutrition in Health and Disease* (15th ed.; Philadelphia: J. B. Lippincott, Co., 1968).
52. Mukai, T., and Howard, J. E.: Some observations on the calcification of rachitic cartilage by urine, Bull. Johns Hopkins Hosp. 112:279, 1963.
53. Nordin, B. E. C., Peacock, M., and Wilkinson, P.: Hypercalcuria and calcium stone disease, Clin. Endocrinol. Metabol. 1:169, 1972.
54. Ogg, C. S.: Dialysis and the treatment of renal failure, Physiotherapy 59:141, 1973.
55. Pak, C. Y. C., Deler, C. S., and Barlter, F. C.: Successful treatment of recurrent nephrolithiasis (calcium stones) with cellular phosphate, N. Engl. J. Med. 290:175, 1974.
56. Pak, C. Y. C., Kaplan, R., Bone, H., Townsend, J., and Waters, O.: A simple test for the diagnosis of absorptive, resorptive and renal hypercalcuria, N. Engl. J. Med. 292:492, 1975.
57. Pandras, J. P.: Dietary management in chronic hemodialysis, Am. J. Clin. Nutr. 21: 638, 1968.
58. Phillips, M. J., and Cooke, J. M. C.: Relation between urinary calcium and sodium in patients with idiopathic hypercalcuria, Lancet 1:1354, 1967.
59. Pinto, B., et al.: Patterns of oxalate metabolism in recurrent oxalate stone formers, Kidney Int. 5:285, 1974.
60. Popovtzer, M. M., Pinggera, W. F., and Robinette, J. B.: Secondary hyperparathyroidism: Conservative management in patients with renal insufficiency, J.A.M.A. 231:960, 1975.
61. Renal stones, magnesium and vitamin B_6 in rats, Nutr. Rev. 19:306, 1961.
62. Robinson, L. G., and Paulbitski, A. H.: Diet therapy and educational program for patients with chronic renal failure, J. Am. Diet. Assoc. 61:531, 1972.
63. Schlotter, L.: What do you teach the dialysis patient? Am. J. Nurs. 70:82, 1970.
64. Schoolwerth, A. C., and Engle, J. E.: Calcium and phosphorus in diet therapy of uremia, J. Am. Diet. Assoc. 66:460, 1975.
65. Simmons, J. M., et al.: Relation of calorie deficiency to growth failure in children on hemodialysis and the growth response to calorie supplementation, N. Engl. J. Med. 285:653, 1971.
66. Slatopolsky, E., Caglan, S., Gradowska, L., et al.: On the prevention of

secondary hyperparathyroidism in experimental renal disease using proportional reduction of dietary phosphorus intake, Kidney Int. 2:147, 1972.
67. Smith, E. B.: Gluten-free breads for patients with uremia, J. Am. Diet. Assoc. 59:572, 1971.
68. Smith, E. B., and Hill, P. A.: Protein in diets of dialyzed and nondialyzed uremic patients, J. Am. Diet. Assoc. 60:389, 1972.
69. Solomons, C. C., and Styner, J.: Osteogenesis imperfecta: Effect of magnesium administration on pyrophosphate metabolism, Calcif. Tissue Res. 3:318, 1969.
70. Sorensen, M. K., and Kopple, J. D.: Assessment of adherence to protein-restricted diets during conservative management of uremia, Am. J. Clin. Nutr. 21:631, 1968.
71. Stein, P. G., and Winn, N. J.: Diet controlled in sodium, potassium, protein and fluid: Use of points for dietary calculation, J. Am. Diet. Assoc. 61:538, 1972.
72. St. Jeor, S. T.: First annual meeting of council on renal nutrition, J. Am. Diet. Assoc. 67:135, 1975.
73. Ulvila, J. M., et al.: Blood pressure in chronic renal failure, J.A.M.A. 220:233, 1972.
74. Vetter, L., and Shapiro, R.: An approach to dietary management of the patient with renal disease, J. Am. Diet. Assoc. 66:158, 1975.
75. Wake, C. J., and Maddock, J. L.: Vitamin-D metabolism in chronic renal failure, Lancet 1:516, 1975.
76. Wang, J.: Conservative management of chronic renal failure, Med. Clin. North Am. 55:137, 1971.
77. Williams, H. E., and Smith, L. H.: Disorders of oxalate metabolism, Am. J. Med. 45:715, 1968.
78. Williams, H. E.: Nephrolithiasis, N. Engl. J. Med. 290:33, 1974.

Chapter 8 / Drug and Nutrient Interactions

CLINICAL MEDICINE has often dealt with the effect of one drug upon the action of another, the so-called drug-drug interactions. However, until recently, little consideration has been given to the effect of drugs upon nutrition, or drug-nutrient interactions. As the number and use of pharmaceutical products increase, the interrelationships between drugs and nutrition become more apparent. Physicians, dietitians and nurses, as well as pharmacists, should become familiar with these interrelationships so that appropriate diets and nutrition can be offered to patients during sickness and convalescence. Drugs can affect taste, appetite, intestinal motility, absorption and metabolism of nutrients. Any interference with the usual intake of food will adversely affect health, and certain foods or patterns of dietary consumption may alter drug absorption and response.

Malnutrition may develop slowly and without prompt recognition from what is thought to be "harmless," long-term drug therapy. Malnutrition may result from misunderstanding or from lack of monitoring of the clinical indicators of nutritional status. For instance, long-term anticonvulsant drug therapy may lead to folate deficiency, osteomalacia and rickets. A rare finding of oral contraceptive therapy is megaloblastic anemia. Cholestyramine resin therapy may cause loss of fat-soluble vitamins, such as vitamin K. Long-term use of glucocorticoids leads to excessive loss of calcium and phosphorus, which may cause osteoporosis. Diuretics, especially the thiazide group, may cause potassium depletion.

Comparison of Drug and Nutrient Absorption

The characteristics of absorption of drugs and nutrients are strikingly different. Absorption of most drugs is governed by lipid solubility, rate of dissociation, pH of medium, particle or molecular size and physical form. Transport across the gastric and/or intestinal mucosa is primarily by passive, nonionic diffusion. Retarded gastric motility produces delayed or reduced absorption of drugs. Absorption is more rapid when drugs are high in concentration. Digestive enzymes and competitive inhibition are not factors in drug absorption.

Absorption of nutrients depends largely on gastrointestinal secre-

151

TABLE 8-1.—SOME CHARACTERISTIC EFFECTS ON ABSORPTION OF
DRUGS AND NUTRIENTS

EFFECT	ABSORPTION OF DRUGS	ABSORPTION OF NUTRIENTS
Lipid solubility	Enhances diffusion of nonionized portion across cell membranes	Important for those nutrients that are lipid-soluble, not those that are water-soluble
pH	Acidic drugs absorbed slowly at low gastric pH	Affects activity of digestive enzymes and solubility of proteins, lipids and electrolytes
Dissociation	When increased, absorption of most drugs reduced	?
Molecular size, shape and form	When increased, absorption reduced	Not as significant; above upper limit in size, absorption is negligible
Route of absorption	Passive, nonionic diffusion mainly; a few have active transport	Nonionic passive diffusion; active transport, pinocytosis and facilitated diffusion
Gastric motility	Absorption of drugs delayed or reduced if GI motility retarded	If GI motility is ↑, absorption ↓
Site of absorption	Stomach or upper intestine	Upper intestine, except for vitamin B_{12}
Digestive enzymes	None	Necessary for proteins, lipids and carbohydrates
Competitive inhibition	None	Described for simple sugars and amino acids

tions, pH and enzyme activity. Transport mechanisms involve passive diffusion, active transport, facilitated diffusion and pinocytosis. The degree of lipid solubility is important only for lipids.[14, 18, 19, 26, 28] A summary of the characteristics of absorption is shown in Table 8-1.

Effects of Drugs on Nutrients

DRUGS AFFECTING GASTRIC AND/OR INTESTINAL MOTILITY.— Mineral oil decreases the absorption of the fat-soluble vitamins A, D, E and K and carotene. Certain cathartics decrease absorption of nutrients. For example, podophyllum jalap and colocynth may cause calcium and potassium loss and steatorrhea. Oxyphenisatin, bisacodyl and phenolphthalein may inhibit intestinal uptake of glucose. Hypertonic solutions of mannitol may injure the absorptive cells, leading to inhibition of transport across the intestinal mucosa of glucose, water and sodium. Chronic and excessive use of some antacids can lead to thiamine deficiency as a result of alkaline destruction of thiamine within the bowel. Certain ganglionic blocking agents and anticholinergics that block or reduce peristalsis lower absorption of some nutrients by decreasing the movement and mixing of intestinal contents. Some of these drugs are methantheline bromide, propantheline bromide and mecamylamine hydrochloride.[5, 18, 19, 26]

HYPOCHOLESTEROLEMIC AGENTS.—Cholestyramine resin, clofibrate and neomycin have been shown to lower serum cholesterol levels. Cholestyramine resin forms unabsorbable complexes with bile acids, preventing their reabsorption and increasing breakdown of cholesterol to bile acids to lower serum cholesterol levels. However, these agents have been associated with a variety of malabsorption phenomena, including malabsorption of vitamin B_{12}, D-xylose, carotene, medium-chain triglycerides, electrolytes, iron, sugar and nitrogen.[18, 19, 26] Table 8–2 gives more explicit details regarding these agents.

SURFACTANTS.—In general, stool softeners or surfactants may affect absorption of nutrients by altering fat dispersion and permeability of the lipoprotein membrane of the mucosal cells. Tween 80 has been shown to improve the absorption of vitamin A in patients with malabsorption syndromes. In an earlier study, Tween 80 was shown to enhance the absorption of neutral fat.[18] Another possibility may be that the surfactant increases the rate of dissolution of solids by increasing the contact between particles and bulk fluid of the gut, leading to an increased amount of drug or nutrient available for absorption. This mechanism is thought to be operative in the action of polysorbate 80 and dioctyl sodium sulfosuccinate.[5]

ANTIMICROBIAL AGENTS.—Para-aminosalicylic acid, neomycin, erythromycin, sulfonamides, broad-spectrum antibiotics—such as the tetracyclines and penicillins—isoniazid, chloramphenicol and others have been implicated as the cause of decreased utilization of folic acid, malabsorption of vitamin B_{12}, decreased bacterial synthesis of vitamin K, impaired absorption of calcium and magnesium, inactivation of pyridoxine and impaired amino acid transfer in protein synthesis.[19, 26] Specifically, para-aminosalicylic acid is associated with impaired vitamin B_{12} absorption, as well as impaired folic acid, iron and cholesterol absorption, because it inhibits absorptive enzymes. Sulfonamides inhibit the bacterial synthesis of folic acid, B vitamins and vitamin K. Tetracyclines chelate with heavy metals and bind with bone calcium. Penicillins inhibit histamine destruction and the hydrolysis of glutathione. Chloramphenicol decreases protein synthesis in systems containing ribonucleic acid and may inhibit amino acid transfer during protein synthesis.[5, 18]
Antibiotic therapy may induce changes in the intestinal flora which

TABLE 8-2.—REPORTED DRUG INTERFERENCES WITH NUTRIENTS

DRUG	INTERFERENCE
Alcohol	Folic acid, vitamin B_{12}, fat ↑ Excretion of magnesium
Analgesics	
Colchicine	Damage to intestinal wall → nonspecific ↓ in absorption ↓ Absorption of vitamin B_{12}, carotene, fat, lactose, D-xylose, electrolytes and cholesterol
Anorexiants	Appetite suppression → growth retardation
Antacids	Alkaline destruction of thiamine → thiamine deficiency; fatty acids
Anticonvulsants	
Barbiturates	Inhibition of absorptive enzymes or ↑ metabolism and turnover → deficiency in body folate and vitamin D ↓ Vitamin B_{12} and D-xylose absorption
Hydantoins	Inhibition of absorptive enzymes ↑ Metabolism and turnover Deficiency in body folate and vitamin D ↑ Urinary excretion of ascorbic acid
Antidepressants	
Tricyclic antidepressants	Stimulation of appetite → weight gain
Antimetabolites	Anti-vitamin action on folic acid
Methotrexate	Damage to intestinal wall → nonspecific ↓ in absorption Inhibition of enzyme system ↓ Vitamin B_{12}, folic acid and D-xylose absorption
Antimicrobials	Appetite suppression and diarrhea → ↓ nutrient absorption
Chloramphenicol	↓ Protein synthesis Altered hemoglobin synthesis → failure of incorporation of Fe into RBC
Isoniazid	Complexation of vitamin B_6 → ↑ excretion of vitamin B_6
Neomycin	See under Hypocholesterolemics
Para-aminosalicylic acid	Inhibition of absorptive enzymes → ↓ vitamin B_{12} absorption, folic acid, iron and cholesterol
Penicillin	Aftertaste with food → suppression of appetite Inhibition of glutathione
Sulfonamides	↓ Synthesis of folic acid, B vitamins and vitamin K
Tetracyclines	Binding of bone calcium ↑ Serum nonprotein N and urinary amino acids and urea
Autonomics	
Ganglionic blockers	↓ Peristalsis → ↓ nutrient absorption
Anticholinergics	Same as above
Cathartics	Malabsorption of protein, calcium, vitamin D and potassium
Bisacodyl	↓ Intestinal uptake of glucose
Colocynth	↑ Loss of calcium, potassium; steatorrhea
Jalap	Same as above
Mannitol	Damage to intestinal wall → ↓ absorption of glucose, water and sodium

154

TABLE 8-2.—*Continued*

DRUG	INTERFERENCE
Oxyphenisatin	↓ Intestinal uptake of glucose
Phenolphthalein	Same as above
Podophyllum	↑ Loss of calcium, potassium; steatorrhea
Chelating agents	Chelation of metals → ↓ absorption of metals
Penicillamine	Complexation of vitamin B_6 → ↑ excretion of vitamin B_6
	↓ Taste acuity and aftertaste → suppression of appetite
Corticosteroids	↓ Glucose tolerance
	↓ Muscle protein
	↑ Liver fat
	↑ Retention of sodium
	↓ Calcium and iron absorption
Diuretics	↑ Excretion of potassium
(except spironolactone and triamterene)	↓ Excretion of potassium
	↓ Excretion of potassium
Hypocholesterolemics	
Cholestyramine resin	↓ Absorption of potassium, fat-soluble vitamins; binds inorganic and hemoglobin Fe in vitro
Clofibrate	↓ Absorption of vitamin B_{12}, D-xylose, carotene, MCT, iron, sugar and electrolytes
	↓ Taste acuity and aftertaste → suppression of appetite
Neomycin	Inactivation of bile acids → ↓ absorption of vitamine B_{12}, lactose, D-xylose, carotene, MCT, iron, sugar, potassium, sodium, calcium and nitrogen
	Damage to intestinal wall
	Steatorrhea
Laxatives	
Mineral oil	↓ Absorption of carotene and vitamins A, D, E and K
Oral contraceptives	Inhibition of absorptive enzymes
	Selective malabsorption or enzyme induction → deficiency in body folate
	↑ Turnover of vitamin B_6 → deficiency in vitamin B_6
	↑ Blood lipids (especially TG)
	↑ Intestinal absorption of iron
Potassium chloride	↓ Absorption of vitamin B_{12}
Sedative-hypnotics	
Glutethimide	↑ Metabolism and turnover of vitamin D → deficiency in vitamin D
	Multivitamin deficiency
Surfactants (stool softeners)	Alteration of fat dispersion and permeability of mucosal cell membrane → alteration of nutrient absorption
Tranquilizers	
Phenothiazines	Stimulation of appetite → weight gain
Chlorpromazine	Hypercholesterolemia

References: 7, 9, 15, 16, 19, 20, 26, 27, 29, 31, 32, and 39.

lead to secondary malabsorption. In addition, antibiotics can increase the number and volume of stools, thereby increasing the amount of undigested food in the feces.

CYTOTOXIC DRUGS.—Methotrexate, aminopterin and other folic acid antagonists are inhibitors of folic acid, interfere with vitamin B_{12} and D-xylose absorption and are responsible for nonspecific changes in the jejunal mucosa. Colchicine is associated with decreased absorption of vitamin B_{12}, carotene, fat and lactose, which is accompanied by increased fecal excretion of nitrogen and electrolytes.[5, 18, 19, 26]

ANTICONVULSANT DRUGS.—Diphenylhydantoin, primidone and phenobarbital appear to impair the utilization of folic acid, vitamin B_{12} and D-xylose. Phenindione induces malabsorption of fat and nitrogen. Other risks of anticonvulsant therapy are osteomalacia and rickets, especially with diphenylhydantoin, primidone and phenytoin. Phenobarbitone has the least effect on serum calcium. The effects of these drugs are secondary to a deficiency in vitamin D and are thought to be related to the increased metabolism and turnover caused by anticonvulsants.[5, 18, 19, 26]

ALCOHOL.—The effects of alcohol on nutritional status and malabsorption of folic acid, vitamin B_{12} and thiamine are well known. In addition, there is increased magnesium excretion. Transient hypomagnesemia has been observed in alcoholic patients undergoing convulsive seizures during acute withdrawal phases.[19, 26]

DIURETICS.—With the exception of triamterene and spironolactone, most diuretics are capable of precipitating serious episodes of hypokalemia through excessive renal clearance of potassium. Thiazides have also been reported to precipitate diabetes.[19, 26]

TABLE 8–3.—MECHANISMS OF DRUG
INTERFERENCE WITH
NUTRITIONAL STATUS

   I. Suppression or stimulation of appetite
  II. Alteration of nutrient absorption
      Alteration of GI transit time
      Alteration of GI pH
      Alteration of bile acid activity
      Alteration of peristalsis
      Inactivation of absorptive enzyme systems
      Competitive inhibition at nutrient's site of absorption
      Damage to absorptive mucosal cells of GI tract
      Complexation of nutrient by drug
 III. Alteration of nutrient's metabolism and utilization
 IV. Alteration of nutrient's excretion

TABLE 8-4.—CATEGORIES OF
DRUGS CAPABLE OF
INTERFERING WITH
NUTRITIONAL STATUS

Antacids
Anorexiants
Anticonvulsants
Antidepressants
Antimicrobials
Appetite stimulants
Autonomic agents
    Anticholinergics
    Ganglionic blockers
Cathartics, laxatives
Corticosteroids
Cytotoxic drugs (folic acid antagonists)
Diuretics
Hypocholesterolemic agents
Oral contraceptives
Surfactants

Many categories of drugs used in treating patients with chronic conditions pose a threat to the patient's nutritional status.

ORAL CONTRACEPTIVES.—Some oral contraceptives have been implicated in impaired folic acid absorption and utilization. The estrogen-progestin combination has been shown to induce biochemical evidence of vitamin B_6 deficiency. Depressed plasma ascorbic acid concentration related to oral contraceptive agents has been suggested.[3, 19, 26]

The reported drug interferences with nutrients can be found in Table 8-2. The mechanisms of drug interference with nutritional status appear in Table 8-3, and the drug categories capable of nutrient interference are listed in Table 8-4.

Effects of Food on Drugs

With the exception of the classics, i.e., tyramine-containing foods and monamine oxidase (MAO) inhibitors or pyridoxine-containing foods and levodopa, relatively few articles in the literature have been devoted to this phenomenon. However, there are four possible means by which drug-food interaction phenomena might occur: (1) the effect of food upon drug absorption; (2) dietary constituents which may alter drug metabolism through enzyme induction or inhibition; (3) foods which may alter the rate of excretion of certain drugs through excessive acidification or alkalinization of urine; and (4) pharmacologically active substances in foods which may alter the response of a drug administered at the same time the food is consumed, e.g., MAO inhibitors and tyramine-containing foods result in an increase in pressor responses. Most of these interactions relate to impaired drug absorption, but the exact mechanisms are poorly understood.[19, 26]

DRUG ADMINISTRATION AND FOOD INGESTION.—Food ingestion reduces the efficiency of absorption of tetracycline, demethylchlortetracycline, chlortetracycline, methacycline, benzathine penicillin G, penicillin V, nafcillin, oxacillin, ampicillin, the erythromycins, triacetyloleandomycin, lincomycin and the sulfonamides. Administration of tetracycline concomitant with intake of dairy products containing large amounts of calcium presumably could result in complex formation of calcium caseinate and impair absorption of the antibiotic. Perhaps more important is the impaired tetracycline absorption with concomitant administration of iron salts, which reduce plasma levels of tetracycline from 10–50%.[19, 26]

Griseofulvin levels are markedly increased after ingestion of a high-fat meal. This could be a significant problem for patients on anticoagulant therapy, since prothrombin time reportedly decreases more when griseofulvin and sodium warfarin (Coumadin) are administered concurrently. Excessive fat intake should be avoided when tetrachloroethylene (used in treating hookworm) is administered to prevent systemic absorption and possible central nervous system toxicity.[19, 26]

A number of drugs are intrinsically irritating to gastric mucosa and should be taken immediately before, with or immediately after meals or with food. The more popular drugs are indomethacin, diphenylhydantoin, phenylbutazone, nitrofurantoin, steroids, metronidazole, iron salts, aminophylline, potassium supplements, aspirin and reserpine.[26]

Mixing drugs with juices and beverages to mask disagreeable taste may precipitate problems regarding acid labile substances, whose absorption may be impaired due to decreased gastric pH or inactivation in acidic media before ingestion. Whole milk is far less acidic than most juices and has a pH range of 6.4 to 6.8. Ampicillin, erythromycin, and penicillin G potassium should not be mixed and/or allowed to stand for any length of time in acidic beverages.[19, 26]

DIETARY CONSTITUENTS AND DRUG METABOLISM.—In the literature, there are many examples of apparent enzyme induction, as well as enzyme inhibition, caused by drugs and their resultant impact on rates of drug metabolism. However, reports of food-induced changes in human drug metabolism have been limited to food contaminants.

Food additives, such as the commonly used anti-oxidants like BHA and butylated hydroxytoluene, are inducers but only at levels far above those in normal use.[21] Pesticide residues, such as DDT, lindane, aldrin and dieldrin, can be found in varying concentrations in all levels of the food chain. These residual concentrations are a function of factors such as the nature of the pest control treatment used in seed preparation, spraying and sprinkling, climate and soil conditioning. Organo-chlorine insecticides absorbed from contaminated food are stored in the body fat and liver of man for prolonged periods of time. However, these accumulations have been considerably below the minimum toxic level. Residual concentrations of certain pesticides have shown some enzyme induction in specific cases.[19, 21, 26]

It has been reported that DDT levels in patients taking phenobarbital and diphenylhydantoin were significantly lower than those in patients who were not taking these drugs. Both of these drugs are known to be microsomal enzyme inducers and, therefore, may act to reduce tissue storage of DDT by this mechanism.[19, 26]

Alcohol interacts with a large number of commonly used drugs: antibiotics, anticoagulants, antihistamines, digitalis, MAO inhibitors, nitroglycerine, diuretics, heavy metals, insulin, iron, puromycin C and others. It specifically interacts with sedatives, opiates, phenothiazines, antidepressants and other psychoactive drugs. Use of alcohol by patients who are taking these drugs should be restricted by the physician.[35] In addition, alcohol stimulates an enzyme-induction process that reduces twofold the biologic half-life of tolbutamide, an oral hypoglycemic agent. This may partially explain the difficulty and high-failure rate of treating "alcoholic-diabetics."[19, 26]

Altering Urinary Excretion Rates.—Changes in urinary pH have altered the excretion rates of some drugs markedly. These alterations are due to the influence of pH on the ionization of weak acids and weak bases. For example, a drug in its nondissociated form diffuses more readily from urine back into blood. The action of acidic drugs is prolonged in acid urine, because a larger proportion of the drug is nondissociated in acid urine than in alkaline urine. In alkaline urine, the drug is primarily an ionized salt. The opposite phenomenon holds for a basic drug, such as amphetamine or quinidine. Changes in diet alone do not easily achieve extreme shifts in urinary pH (below 5.0 and above 8.0). However, increased urinary acidification or alkalinization occur with concomitant ingestion of acid or alkaline-ash diets and urinary acidifiers (ammonium chloride, ascorbic acid, mandelamine) or alkalinizers (carbonic anhydrase inhibitors, bicarbonate or citrate solution). Extreme shifts in urinary pH can have important clinical significance, as described in a case of quinidine intoxication. The patient consumed antacids and an alkaline-ash diet daily, which produced alkaline urine and decreased quinidine excretion during maintenance therapy with quinidine. This culminated in a serious arrhythmia requiring hospitalization of the patient.[19, 26]

PHARMACOLOGICALLY ACTIVE SUBSTANCES PRESENT IN FOODS. — One of the most frequently discussed interactions is that which occurs between tyramine-containing foods and MAO inhibitors. A group of naturally occurring constituents called pressor amines — histamine, tyramine, tryptamine, tyrosine and their metabolites, such as serotonin and norepinephrine — cause vasoconstriction and a rise in blood pressure when consumed by patients taking MAO inhibitors. The MAO inhibitors are antidepressant drugs, including isocarboxazid (Marplan), tranylcypromine (Parnate), pargyline hydrochloride (Eutonyl), phenelzine sulfate (Nardil), and nialamide (Niamid). The hypertensive syndrome reported in this food-drug interaction has been described as similar to that seen in pheochromocytoma — headache, fever and hypertension. However, most of the food-drug attacks have occurred ½ to 2 hours after patients have eaten certain cheeses.[5, 19, 26] Table 8–5 lists foods high in tyramine which should be avoided by patients who are receiving MAO inhibitors.

The vitamin B_6 (pyridoxine) content of food seems to be an important factor influencing the activity of levodopa. This vitamin has been shown to potentiate the vasopressor effect of injected levodopa. Pyridoxine apparently stimulates increased activity of the dopa-decarboxylase enzyme in the liver and peripheral tissues. Therefore, there is an increased rate of dopamine formation from levodopa in the periphery. Since dopamine that is not formed in the brain cannot cross the blood-brain barrier, symptoms of Parkinson's disease are not alleviated. It has been reported that the usual amount of pyridoxine contained in a standard daily diet would not interfere with the therapeutic effect of levodopa.[5]

When ingested in excessive amounts, true licorice, not synthetic licorice flavor, can cause hypokalemia, salt and water retention, hypertension and alkalosis. The glycyrrhizinic acid in licorice is similar to desoxycorticosterone. Chronic excessive consumption of imported licorice may be contraindicated, therefore, in patients on cardiac glycosides, nonpotassium-sparing diuretics and low salt diets.[5, 19, 26]

Monosodium L-glutamate (MSG), a widely used food additive, has been implicated as the causative agent of the "Chinese restaurant syndrome." Symptoms of the Chinese restaurant syndrome include headache, burning sensations in the extremities, facial pressure and chest-pain mimicking angina. The pharmacologic effects of MSG appear to be dose related, and the threshold dose tremendously varies from one person to the next. Apparently, MSG causes transient hypernatremia. Patients on long-term diuretic therapy should be cautioned about consuming large quantities of Won Ton soup and other Chinese foods containing MSG.[19, 26, 34]

TABLE 8-5.—FOODS HIGH IN TYRAMINE THAT
SHOULD NOT BE TAKEN WITH MONOAMINE
OXIDASE INHIBITORS*

FOOD	TYRAMINE (μG/GM OR μG/ML)
Cheese	
Boursalt	?
Brick	?
Brie	180
Camembert	86
Cheddar, N.Y. State	1416
Ermantaler	225
Gruyere	516
Mozzarella	?
Stilton blue	466
Yeast extracts (depends on brand)	
Marmite	?
Alcoholic drinks (depends on brand)	
Beer	1.8–4.4
Wine: Sherry	3.6
Chianti	25.4
Fruits and vegetables (and their juices)	
Bananas	
Broad beans (contain dopa or dopamine)	
Passion fruit	
Pineapples	
Plantains	
Other possible agents	
Beef livers (fresh)	5.4
Chicken livers (fresh)	0.5
Chocolate (depends on fermentation time of cacao bean; contains catecholamine derivative, vanillin)	
Pickled herring	3030
Yogurt, coffee, cola (caffeine-containing drinks)	

*MAO inhibitors: isocarboxazid—Marplan (Roche); pargyline—Eutonyl (Abbott); phenelzine—Nardil (Warner-Chilcott); tranylcypromine—Parnate (SmithKline).
References: 5, 16, and 26.

TABLE 8–6.—MECHANISMS OF FOOD
INTERFERENCE WITH DRUG THERAPY

I. Alteration of absorption of orally administered drugs
   Alteration of GI transit time and motility
   Alteration of GI secretions and pH
   Alteration of osmolality of GI tract
   Alteration of ionization of drug
   Alteration of stability of drug
   Alteration of solubility of drug
   Complexation of drug by dietary component
II. Alteration of drug's distribution
III. Alteration of drug's metabolism
IV. Alteration of drug's excretion
V. Exertion of agonistic or antagonistic pharmacologic
   response by active substance in food

A summary of the mechanisms of food interference with drug therapy appears in Table 8–6.

Drug Effects on Taste and Appetite

Several drugs have been reported as the cause of hypogeusesthesia (decreased taste acuity) or dysgeusia (unpleasant or altered taste sensation). These agents are griseofulvin, penicillamine, clofibrate, lincomycin, 5-mercaptopyridoxal, phenindione, oxyphedrin hydrochloride and some tranquilizers. In addition, streptomycin may cause a metallic taste in the mouth. Because of altered taste sensation and loss of appetite, treatment with these drugs might lead to decreased food intake and ultimately to malnutrition. Excessive use of cytotoxic and unpleasant-tasting drugs, such as chloral hydrate, paraldehyde, vitamin B complex and uncoated penicillin preparations, may also cause loss of appetite.[26, 40]

Bulk agents, such as methylcellulose (celevac, cellucon) and guar gum (Decorpa) have a slight effect on reducing appetite. They take up fluid and swell in the stomach to give patients a feeling of fullness. Amphetamines and their related compounds are known to be effective anorectic agents but may become addictive and have numerous side effects. Biguanides, oral hypoglycemic agents (Phenformain and Metformin), may reduce appetite and food intake. When injected, glucagon does the same.[25]

Appetite improvement and weight gain have been seen in patients using psychotropic agents, such as the phenothiazines, benzodiazepines and tricyclic antidepressants. These effects may be secondary to altered mental status. Alcohol, when taken in a small amount before a meal, increases the appetite by stimulating sense of taste, increasing flow of saliva and gastric and pancreatic secretions. Insulin-induced hypoglycemia is associated with increased appetite. Androgens and anabolic steroids, like norethandrolone (Nilevar), methandienone (Dienabol) and nandrolone phenpropionate (Durabolin), exert slight effects on appetite. In addition, corticotrophin and some glucocorticoids, such as cortisone, increase appetite in man. The sulphonylureas (oral antidiabetic agents), especially tolbutamide, chlorpropamide, tolazamide, glibenclamide, acetohexamide and pyrimidine-glymidine, may increase appetite and weight gain by stimulating release of pancreatic insulin.[6, 25, 26, 40]

Drugs and Special Diets

We seldom give enough thought or attention to drugs as part of the diet or foods as part of the drug regimen. However, a physician may write an order for a special diet, e.g., a low sodium diet, in the course of treatment of a cardiac patient. The dietitian spends considerable time preparing a diet to meet the specific medical needs of the patient, as well as his psychosocial needs. The pharmacist may not be notified of all the patient's needs and may dispense a medication high in sodium, which could cause a serious problem. A similar situation might happen if a renal patient who requires a potassium-restricted diet is given a salt substitute that is high in potassium. This commonly occurs with diabetics who receive a large glucose load in cough syrup.

It behooves all members of the health care team to become involved in a patient's "total medical care." This, then, means that the physician, dietitian and pharmacist, as well as the nurse directly involved in patient care, must become familiar with the sodium content of drugs; the potassium content of drugs, foods and salt substitutes; and sugar-free medications.[11, 13]

Summary

Patients on long-term and multiple-drug regimens are more apt to develop drug-induced nutritional deficiency states. A physician should not prescribe long-term drug therapy without careful monitoring of the nutritional status of his patients and should give nutritional supplements as required.[33]

There are drugs we would like to have in nutrition. As Raisz stated, "It is easy to imagine wonder-drugs for nutritional and metabolic disease: drugs that would dissolve the collagen in cirrhosis, remove atherosclerotic plaques, count calories in the intestinal lumen, and stop absorption at a given number, reverse transport to secrete nutrients for weight loss, or let us turn metabolism off or on at will to maintain a desired blood alcohol concentration." Then, because of their adverse effects, Raisz listed drugs we wish we could eliminate from nutrition: alcohol, amphetamines, xanthines, cigarettes, marijuana, LSD, sedatives, tranquilizers and narcotics.[30] However, these views are somewhat unrealistic. We must continue to be aware of drug nutrient interactions so they may be dealt with intelligently.

REFERENCES

1. Berman, H. A., and Weinstein, L.: Antibiotics and nutrition, Am. J. Clin. Nutr. 24:260, 1971.
2. Boots, L., Cornwell, P. E., and Beck, L. R.: Effect of ethynodiol diacetate and mestranol on serum folic acid and vitamin B_{12} levels and on tryptophan metabolism in baboons, Am. J. Clin. Nutr. 28:354, 1975.
3. Butterworth, C. E., Jr.: Interactions of nutrients with oral contraceptives and other drugs, J. Am. Diet. Assoc. 62:510, 1973.
4. Butterworth, C. E., Jr.: The dimensions of clinical nutrition, Am. J. Clin. Nutr. 28:943, 1975.
5. Carmichael, B. L.: Some aspects of diet and its relationship to drug therapy, Can. J. Hosp. Pharm. 202–209, 1973.
6. Carson, J. S., and Gormican, A.: Disease-medication relationships in altered taste sensitivity, J. Am. Diet. Assoc. 68:550, 1976.
7. Christakis, G., and Miridjanian, A.: Diets, drugs, and their interrelationships, J. Am. Diet. Assoc. 52:21, 1968.
8. Dickerson, J. W. T., and Walker, R.: Nutrition, age and drug metabolism, Proc. Nutr. Soc. 33:191, 1974.
9. Eisenstein, A.: Effects of adrenal cortical hormones on carbohydrate, protein, and fat metabolism, Am. J. Clin. Nutr. 26:113, 1973.
10. Fineberg, S. K.: The sensible management of obesity with diet and drugs, Drug Therapy, 3:32, 1973.
11. Fish, K. H., and Pearson, R. E.: Sodium content of selected medicines, Hosp. Pharm. 5:5, 1970.
12. Gray, G. M.: Drugs, malnutrition, and carbohydrate absorption, Am. J. Clin. Nutr. 26:121, 1973.
13. Goldschmidt, L. A., and Durgin, J. M., Sr.: Drugs and special diets, Hosp. Pharm. 7:15, 1972.
14. Goodman, L. S., and Gilman, A. (ed.): *The Pharmacological Basis of Therapeutics* (5th ed.; New York: Macmillan Publishing Co., Inc., 1975).
15. Greenberger, N. J.: Effects of antibiotics and other agents on the intestinal transport of iron, Am. J. Clin. Nutr. 26:104, 1973.
16. Hethcox, J. M., and Stanaszek, W. F.: Interactions of drugs and diet, Hosp. Pharm. 9:373, 1974.
17. Hodges, R. E.: Nutrition and the pill, J. Am. Diet. Assoc. 59:212, 1971.
18. Krondl, A.: Present understanding of the interactions of drugs and food during absorption, Can. Med. Assoc. J. 103:360, 1970.
19. Lambert, M. L.: Drug and diet interactions, Am. J. Nurs. 75:402, 1975.

20. Longstreth, G. F., and Newcomer, A. D.: Drug-induced malabsorption, Mayo Clin. Proc. 50:284, 1975.
21. McLean, A. E. M.: Molecules in food that alter drug metabolism, Proc. Nutr. Soc. 33:197, 1974.
22. Marks, V.: Effect of drugs on carbohydrate metabolism, Proc. Nutr. Soc. 33:209, 1974.
23. Mayer, J.: Iatrogenic malnutrition, Postgrad. Med. 49:247, 1971.
24. Mehta, S., et al.: Chloramphenicol metabolism in children, Am. J. Clin. Nutr. 28:977, 1975.
25. Pawan, G. L. S.: Drugs and appetite, Proc. Nutr. Soc. 33:239, 1974.
26. Pierpaoli, P. G.: Drug therapy and diet, Drug Intellig. Clin. Pharm. 6:89, 1972.
27. Poskitt, E. M. E.: Clinical problems related to the use of drugs in malnutrition, Proc. Nutr. Soc. 33:203, 1974.
28. Prescott, L. F.: Gastrointestinal absorption of drugs, Med. Clin. North Am. 58:907, 1974.
29. Rahman, F., and Cain, G. D.: Intestinal malabsorption due to drugs, Drug Therapy 4:123, 1974.
30. Raisz, L. G.: Some drugs we would like to have in nutrition and metabolism, Am. J. Clin. Nutr. 26:125, 1973.
31. Reynolds, E. H.: Iatrogenic nutritional effects of anticonvulsants, Proc. Nutr. Soc. 33:225, 1974.
32. Roe, D. A.: Drug-induced vitamin deficiencies, Drug Therapy 3:23, 1973.
33. Roe, D. A.: Nutritional side effects of drugs, Food Nutr. News 45:1, 1973.
34. Schaumburg, H. H., et al.: Monosodium L-glutamate: Its pharmacology and role in the Chinese restaurant syndrome, Science 163:826, 1969.
35. Seixas, F. A.: Alcohol and its drug interactions, Ann. Intern. Med. 83:86, 1975.
36. Smith, J. L., Goldsmith, G. A., and Lawrence, J. D.: Effects of oral contraceptive steroids on vitamin and lipid levels in serum, Am. J. Clin. Nutr. 28:371, 1975.
37. Streiff, R. R.: Folate deficiency and oral contraceptives, J.A.M.A. 214:105, 1970.
38. Truswell, A. S.: Drugs and lipid metabolism, Proc. Nutr. Soc. 33:215, 1974.
39. Wilson, C. W. M.: Vitamins and drug metabolism with particular reference to vitamin C, Proc. Nutr. Soc. 33:231, 1974.
40. Yosselson, S.: Drugs and nutrition, Drug Intellig. Clin. Pharm. 10:8, 1976.

Index